PAIN RECOVERY

How to Find Balance and Reduce Suffering from Chronic Pain

A Comprehensive Opioid-Free Approach

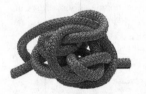

Mel Pohl, MD, FASAM

Frank J. Szabo, Jr., LADC

Daniel Shiode, Ph.D.

Robert Hunter, Ph.D.

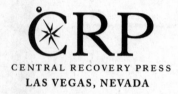

CENTRAL RECOVERY PRESS
LAS VEGAS, NEVADA

CENTRAL RECOVERY PRESS

Central Recovery Press (CRP) is committed to publishing exceptional material addressing addiction treatment, recovery, and behavioral health care, including original and quality books, audio/visual communications, and Web-based new media. Through a diverse selection of titles, it seeks to impact the behavioral health care field with a broad range of unique resources for professionals, recovering individuals, and their families. For more information, visit www.centralrecoverypress.com.

Central Recovery Press, Las Vegas, NV 89129
© 2009 by Central Recovery Press, Las Vegas, NV

ISBN-13: 978-0-9799869-9-4
ISBN-10: 0-9799869-9-0

16 15 14 13 12 11 10   2 3 4 5

Publisher: Central Recovery Press
             3371 N Buffalo Drive
             Las Vegas, NV 89129

Cover design and interior by Sara Streifel, Think Creative Design

To all the courageous clients and their families
who participated in the Chronic Pain Rehabilitation Program
at Las Vegas Recovery Center.

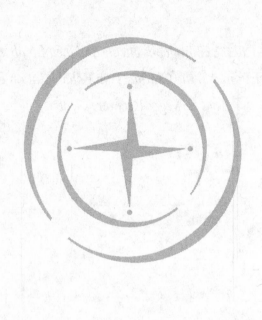

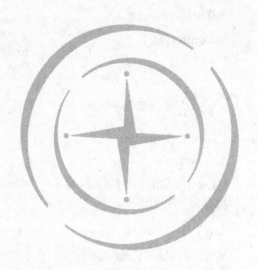

CHAPTER NINE

CHAPTER TEN

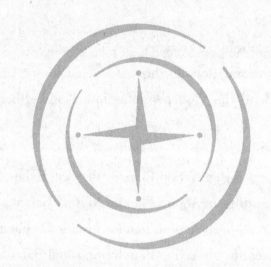

PREFACE

Pain Recovery: How to Find Balance and Reduce Suffering from Chronic Pain is a collaborative effort based on our multidisciplinary knowledge and professional experience treating clients with chronic pain and addiction in the Chronic Pain Rehabilitation Program at Las Vegas Recovery Center (LVRC).

While researching the outcome data and readmission assessments of our addiction treatment program, we found that chronic pain was a common denominator for a large percentage of clients who returned to treatment because of relapse. These clients were motivated for recovery and had successfully completed treatment, but ended up relapsing after seeking traditional pain management to deal with their chronic pain. Most of these clients reported relapsing with prescribed medication (alcohol was often involved as well). They were not able to take the prescribed medication without problems—their use of opioids in an attempt to eliminate their pain resulted in relapse. In other words, they were unable to reconcile their recovery with taking pain medications to treat their pain.

To meet the needs of these clients and others like them, the Chronic Pain Rehabilitation Program was created. After treating more than 100 clients with chronic pain, we realized that the concept of recovery was new to many of them. These clients believed the only issue that needed to be addressed was their physical pain. The more we learned about pain, the more aware we became of the importance of treating all the factors that contribute to the total experience of pain.

From this body of clinical work evolved the concept of pain recovery— a multidimensional approach to treating chronic pain that addresses the physical, mental, emotional, and spiritual aspects of pain, as well as problematic use of medications and addiction.

We have consolidated these concepts, our experience, clients' input, and the fundamentals of the Chronic Pain Rehabilitation Program into a workbook format that is accessible to anyone affected by chronic pain. The book is also designed to be a useful tool for clinicians who treat people with chronic pain. Our intention in writing this book is to offer an empowering, interactive guide that promotes the treatment of chronic pain in a holistic manner without mood-altering drugs.

Mel Pohl, MD, FASAM • Frank J. Szabo, Jr., LADC
Daniel Shiode, Ph.D. • Robert Hunter, Ph.D.

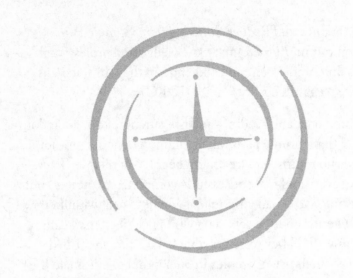

ACKNOWLEDGEMENTS

We would like to express our deepest appreciation and gratitude to Stuart Smith for having faith in us and providing an opportunity for us to utilize our experience, strength, and hope to help others discover pain recovery. Stuart's vision, commitment, and dedication made this book possible.

To our supportive families and friends who make the work we do possible.

To the contributors who allowed us to share their stories of how to live with grace and courage as they walked on the path of pain recovery.

To the excellent editorial staff at Central Recovery Press: Nancy Schenck, Dan Mager, Daniel Kaelin, and Helen O'Reilly. And, especially to Valerie Killeen, for the expert job she did editing this book.

To the skilled and dedicated clinical team and support staff at Las Vegas Recovery Center.

To Sara Streifel, Think Creative Design, for designing this book. To David Fulk for proofreading.

We also would like to thank Denise Crosson and Sarah Batchelor for their contributions.

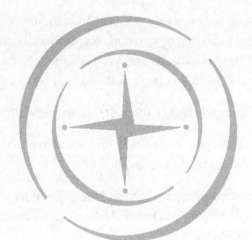

INTRODUCTION

If you suffer from chronic pain and pain medications are not working for you, this book was created to help you. At a time when the medical field is moving further toward management of pain with prescription drugs and procedures, we have developed a tool for those with problematic use of medication or other substances.

Pain Recovery: How to Find Balance and Reduce Suffering from Chronic Pain offers a way to live comfortably, with some sense of ease, and free from habit-forming substances. You will learn how to develop healthy thinking about your pain, minimize suffering by addressing the emotional aspects of chronic pain, ease physical discomfort by applying adjunctive therapies and techniques, and restore well-being by developing your spirituality. In other words, you will learn how to find balance in your life, including your experience of pain.

Some of you may not identify with recovery because it's a term that is traditionally associated with addiction. In this book we will define recovery as the process of moving from imbalance to balance. If you do not feel you are an addict, don't let that interfere with the process. This method works just as well for those who are addicted to medication as for those who don't identify as addicts but who are not getting positive results from their pain-management program.

Pain recovery will require that you try new techniques and be open to thinking differently about your pain. So in order to get the most benefit out of this book, we encourage you to let go of any preconceived notions, put your trust in the process, and proceed with an open mind.

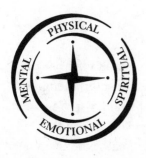

The Four Points of Balance

Pain recovery is grounded in balancing the individual: 1) physically, 2) mentally, 3) emotionally, and 4) spiritually. The four points of balance provide a framework for you to use to identify the areas where imbalance has caused unmanageability in your life and with your family. These points are, of course, interconnected.

To find recovery, you must pay attention to every point of this model (see diagram) and the effect each has on the others. Additionally, your relationships and actions are a reflection of your internal state of balance. Chronic pain is a manifestation of imbalance, typically physical, but, as you will learn, also mental, emotional, and spiritual. Developing an awareness of the points and applying the necessary corrections to bring them back into balance is where the solutions to chronic pain and other life challenges lie. As a result of finding balance in pain recovery, your pain level will diminish.

Overview

Part One includes four chapters that explore chronic pain, addiction, and pain recovery to provide you with a foundation of knowledge and allow you to assess your particular situation. Chapter One explains the causes, characteristics, and effects of chronic pain. In Chapter Two we delve into the complex and sensitive subject of addiction. Chapter Three asks you to examine your use of pain medication and other substances and consider the possibility that you have addiction. Chapter Four explains pain recovery and the four points of balance in detail.

Part Two includes four chapters—one devoted to each of the points—that will help you discover the areas where imbalance is contributing to your negative experience of pain and teach you ways to rebalance them, thus decreasing pain and reducing suffering.

Part Three focuses on your recovery. Once you have identified where you are out of balance, you will be ready to take action and implement changes. Chapter Nine will address your relationships and emphasize the importance of giving and receiving support for recovery to be successful. Chapter Ten deals with actions and gives you an opportunity to create your own action plan for each of the four points to continually bring them back into balance. Lastly, a focused, long-term care plan is provided to help you proactively stay in the pain-recovery process.

To reinforce these concepts, throughout the book we have included the personal stories of individuals who have been and continue to be successful in pain recovery. They have shared, in their own words, their experiences with chronic pain, addiction, and recovery in an effort to help others who are struggling.

How to Use This Book

This book is designed for you to write in, highlight, take notes on, and refer back to. It may be helpful for you to share portions of your work with a counselor, therapist, family member, close friend, sponsor, and/or other professional health care provider. Although each chapter is written to stand on its own, we suggest you start at the beginning and do not skip any chapters. Pace yourself and take breaks when you need to. If you find yourself stuck or having difficulty with an exercise, do not stop working; rather, move on to the next exercise and come back later to the one you are having difficulty with. Don't be afraid to ask for help along the way.

One of the purposes of this book is to help you conceive of a life free from the medications that have been creating problems for you. For those of you who successfully get off medications, be prepared for the likelihood that as they leave your system and the anesthetic effects wear off, your emotions and physical pain will intensify. This is only temporary, since you may feel things you have been numb to for years. Chronic pain has probably affected you for a long time, so be patient and expect a miracle, but don't expect the miracle to happen overnight and don't stop the journey before the miracle happens. Stay positive and hopeful that you *will* experience lasting improvement in your pain level without addictive substances, and begin to live in a more functional and comfortable way.

Now your journey of pain recovery begins, and it is time to go to work.

Important Information about Discontinuing Medications

CAUTION: Do not simply stop your medications. Over time, your body may have become accustomed to them and may be physically dependent on them. You must consult a knowledgeable health care provider or treatment center to supervise withdrawal from habit-forming medications, including opioids, sedatives, hypnotics, and alcohol. Stopping these medications suddenly may be dangerous.

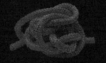

Part I

EXPLORE

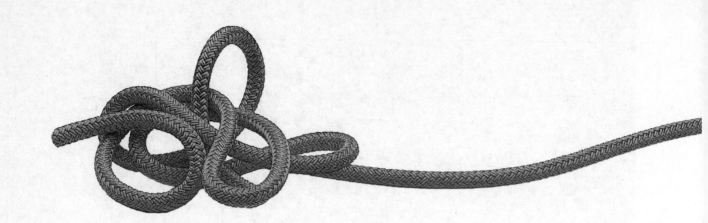

Chronic Pain: An Overview

Pain is an intriguing phenomenon, the source of consternation, irritation, and suffering for millions since the beginning of time. It alerts us that something is wrong—that there is damage or threat of damage to our tissues. Pain is usually produced at the site of an injury and is processed in our complex, computer-like nervous system, causing a vast array of physical and emotional responses. The simplest response is to withdraw from the source of pain and then to protect the area that hurts.

Pain occurs in the body as a result of the interaction of nerve cells, the spinal cord, and the brain (together known as the nervous system). Interactions of a multitude of chemicals, including endorphins, prostaglandins, and neurotransmitters, with electrical impulses coming from the nerve cells create the pain experience, and also pain relief. The brain is exquisitely complex. The part of the brain that processes pain impulses, mainly the thalamus, interacts with other areas of the brain that govern memory, emotions, alertness, movement, blood pressure, hormone levels, and hundreds of other functions. The net effect, in a split second—a composite result of many inputs and outputs—is the experience of pain. Needless to say, this system is efficient beyond that of the most sophisticated computer; however, in the case of chronic pain, the system has gone awry.

Acute and Chronic Pain

There are two types of pain, acute and chronic. In acute pain, the computer functions properly, as it was meant to. With chronic pain, on the other hand, it is as if the computer has been affected by a nasty virus, turning previously healthy and needed mechanisms into overactive and inefficient impulses that disrupt normal function.

Acute pain is time-limited—usually gone within a few hours to days. It may last weeks to a few months, but it eventually goes away. Acute pain can be associated with fractured bones, sore teeth, bruises, cuts, surgeries and their aftermath, infections, and a variety of other injuries and conditions. It exists when there has been damage, and as the damage heals, the pain subsides and eventually resolves, and life returns to the way it was before. Acute pain is part of your body's "response-to-injury" system, which causes you to try to put an end to the offending, pain-causing experience. You also learn from painful experiences and are less likely to do something that causes pain (although later as we explain addiction, you will see that this is not true in all cases).

Chronic pain continues beyond three to six months and has outlived any useful function. It should have gone away, but persists. It is the exaggerated response of the nervous system to damage, but also to other conditions and situations that occur in the brain. It is often pain out of proportion to the prior injury or damage. Sometimes a condition will develop for no apparent reason, and there is not even a clear physical basis for the protracted pain. This is not to say that the pain is in any way unreal or imagined. Some people's bodies simply respond differently over time to certain conditions, damage, or injury. The result is pain that won't quit.

Chronic pain is pain that continues beyond three to six months, has outlived any useful function, and may or may not have a clear physical basis.

That's the worst news about chronic pain—though it may wax and wane, in most cases it doesn't go away. Twenty-five percent of the US population is affected by chronic pain, according to estimates from the National Center for Health Statistics. It is one of the major reasons people go to doctors. As we age, there is a greater chance we will hurt as a result of damaging events, wear-and-tear, and deteriorating conditions.

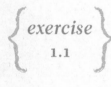

{ exercise }

1.1

Types of Chronic Pain _____

Here is just a partial list of the many potential causes of chronic pain. Find the cause(s) of your pain and check it/them off or write them in the space provided if the causes are not listed.

____ Back, neck, and joint pain, which can result from tension, muscle injury, nerve damage, disc disease, or arthritis.

____ Burn pain, which can continue long after a burn wound has healed.

_____ Chronic pelvic pain, which refers to any pain in your pelvic region (the area between your belly button and your hips) from tumors, infections, or scar tissue.

_____ Cancer pain, which can result from the growth of a tumor with pressure on nerves, from treatment of the disease (chemotherapy or radiation treatments), or from other effects on the body.

_____ Infections that didn't respond to treatment, which can occur almost anywhere in the body.

_____ Chronic abdominal pain (with or without physical explanation or findings), ulcers, gallbladder disease, pancreatitis, or gastroesophageal reflux disease (GERD).

_____ Inflammatory bowel disease, irritable bowel syndrome, or other intestinal problems.

_____ Bursitis, which can affect any joint, most commonly knees, shoulders, hips, elbows, or wrists.

_____ Head and facial pain, which can be caused by dental problems, temporomandibular joint (TMJ) disorders, trigeminal neuralgia, or conditions affecting the nerves in the face.

_____ Chronic headaches, such as migraines, cluster headaches, and tension headaches.

_____ Multiple sclerosis, which can include numbness, aching, or pain.

_____ Angina or chest pain from heart disease.

_____ Uterine fibroid tumors (growths in the womb that can be associated with bleeding).

_____ Chronic obstructive pulmonary disease (COPD) or emphysema.

_____ Peripheral vascular disease (inadequate blood circulation to arms and legs).

_____ Ankylosing spondylitis (severe arthritis with restriction of spinal movement).

_____ Myofascial pain syndromes (heightened experience of pain coming from the brain, which impacts soft tissue and muscles). This includes fibromyalgia, which is characterized by tenderness in multiple trigger points, widespread muscle pain, fatigue, and stiffness.

_____ Whiplash that doesn't go away after an accident.

_____ Broken bones that healed incompletely or in the wrong position.

____ Arthritis (rheumatoid, osteo-, or other forms), which can affect any joint, including hips, knees, neck, back, fingers, wrists, and feet.

____ Neuropathy from a variety of conditions, including HIV/AIDS, injury, and cancer.

____ Other: _____

_____

_____

_____

ALL PAIN IS REAL

Since chronic pain frequently cannot be seen or measured, unlike a broken arm (acute pain), doctors, colleagues, friends, or family may question or doubt your pain. In effect, it doesn't matter if anyone believes you, but it is extremely important for you to acknowledge that *all pain is real.* Your nervous system is made up of electrical circuits modified by chemical neurotransmitters, and the sum total of how these billions of cells interact is your essence—your joy, fear, sight, smell, and all sensations, and your experience of pain.

Pain Is a Subjective, Personal Experience

For some people chronic pain can be disabling, while for others it is merely annoying. Just as pain is entirely subjective, your responses to pain and the responses of your family may vary widely. Some of you stay in bed when you hurt; some of you go about your business. Your unique experience of pain is based on many personal factors, including:

✿ Age.	✿ Gender.
✿ Ethnicity.	✿ Culture.
✿ Religion.	✿ Environment.
✿ Circumstances (context).	✿ Attitudes.
✿ Stereotypes.	✿ Social influences.
✿ Prior experience with pain.	✿ Hormone levels.

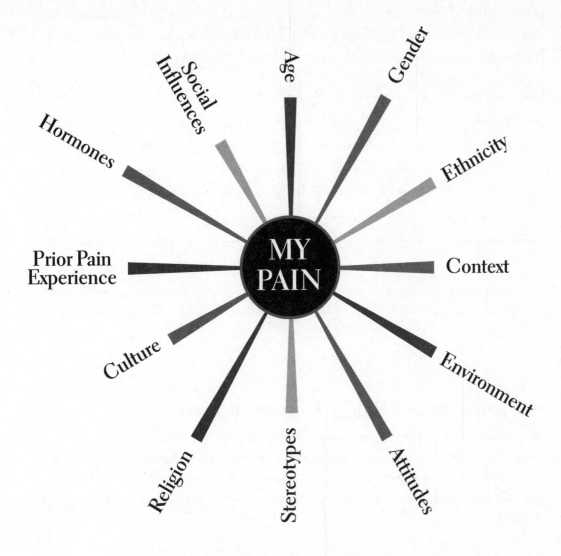

There are countless examples of how these factors can influence your perception of pain. For instance, studies have identified a number of gender differences regarding pain perception. Women are likely to experience pain more often and with greater intensity, while men are less likely to seek help for and express their pain. Attitudes toward and expressions of pain also vary among different cultures. For example, Western cultures tend to have a much lower threshold for pain than some Asian cultures where pain is viewed as having spiritual meaning. If you have had a prior painful experience, you might expect this occurrence to go similarly, and that will affect your actions and, in turn, your pain.

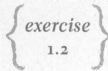

exercise
1.2

Pain Is Subjective_____

Describe how your experience of pain has been affected by the personal factors previously listed or list other factors you believe affected your pain.

_____

_____

_____

_____

_____

_____

_____

_____

_____

_____

_____

Secondary Gain: A Hidden Barrier to Recovery

Secondary gain refers to any perceived benefit you receive from having pain. If not identified, secondary gain gives you unconscious reasons for holding onto your pain. This does not mean you are pretending to hurt for the benefits you get, just that the perceived benefits make the pain rewarding in some ways and thus more complicated to treat.

Some examples of secondary gain that might result from having chronic pain include:

- Receiving more attention.

- Not having to work.

- Being excused from responsibilities.

- Being on disability—essentially, being paid to be in pain.

- Getting out of activities.

- Having an excuse to take medication.

You may view secondary gain as deserved compensation for the pain you experience. These thought processes may be conscious or totally unconscious. Either way, if these beliefs remain unexamined, they may interfere with your ability to improve your condition. Taking inventory of secondary gain you may be experiencing and examining your attitudes about this is an important step in moving toward balance.

In the preface of *A Day without Pain*, Mel Pohl, MD, recounts the role of secondary gain in his personal story of chronic pain:

> *Much as I hate to admit it, in some odd way, the pain I was experiencing and the consequences of having that pain served a function in my life. Actually, the pain had some surprising advantages for me. I didn't realize it at the time, but because of my pain I didn't have to exercise. I had a great excuse to sit around and watch TV, and, of course I had to eat while I was watching TV, which gave me an acceptable excuse for gaining weight. After all, I was in pain. In most of my conversations with friends and family, the opening line usually was "How's your back?" A well-timed groan or moan, more often than not, elicited the sought-after sympathetic "poor Melly…"*

> *Now at the time, if you told me that any of this served me, I would have slugged you. After all, I was hurting, frustrated, furious, and miserable a good part of the time. I felt helpless, powerless, and hopeless. How could anyone suggest I was benefiting from my pain? Thankfully, not a soul dared to make such a suggestion. Without question this would have been a good reason to bite some heads off. I needed an excuse to yell and scream. As long as I stayed angry, my muscles stayed tight. The harder I tried to be powerful and overcome the pain, the more powerless and in pain I was. The more I resisted, the worse I hurt.*

> *Today my pain is still there, but it is much less. What changed? My attitude. I experience my pain in an entirely different way. I got tired of the pain, of complaining, and of being miserable. I realized that my identity was my back pain, and I had become locked in the cycle of the futile search for freedom from suffering. By my resisting, paradoxically, the hurt got worse. I learned to stop fighting and judging the pain. And, lo and behold, it disappeared—often for days at a time.*

> *One of the insights I gained was that I was experiencing something known as secondary gain. In other words, I was gaining something (attention, sympathy, support, an excuse for my inactivity) from my negative or maladaptive behaviors. Furthermore, as I gave up my resistance, I found freedom.*

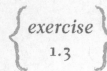

{ *exercise*
1.3 }

Secondary Gain _____

List all the real and perceived benefits you have ever received from having chronic pain. Be sure to include the things you get, as well as things you were or are able to avoid. One example of each is provided for thought.

PHYSICAL

{example: I don't have to help around the house.}

SOCIAL

{example: If I don't show up or cancel at the last minute, everyone understands.}

EMOTIONAL

{example: If I get frustrated or angry, I can blame it on my pain.}

FAMILIAL

(include emotional, as well as specific household or practical responsibilities)

{example: My family pays more attention to me when my pain is bad.}

WORK LIFE

{example: If I call in sick, I can always say it's because of my pain.}

FINANCIAL

{example: I receive workers' compensation payments. It's less money than I made when I worked, but enough to live on. I can't do the same job, so why should I take a job that pays less?}

SEXUAL

{example: My partner no longer expects me to work as hard at providing him or her with sexual pleasure.}

It's important to look closely at secondary gain, as the perceived benefits might not be as attractive as you believe. Most of the time secondary gain is not gain at all, but loss. Chronic pain sufferers often inadvertently buy into secondary gain without looking at primary loss.

Most people find they are just stuck and afraid to move forward. Once you walk through this fear, you will find you gain much more by a return to normalcy in your life.

Examining Secondary Gain _____ {*exercise* 1.4}

Go over the list of examples of secondary gain you identified and take a minute to look at what is actually going on. Write about your observations.

_____

_____

_____

_____

_____

_____

_____

Manifestations of Chronic Pain

Chronic pain can be a troublesome annoyance or a devastating curse that interrupts life functions, relationships, employment, and most things that bring us satisfaction. It takes over our lives, consumes us, and threatens our well-being and the well-being of those who care about us—family, friends, coworkers.

For many with chronic pain, and probably most of you who are reading this, traditional pain management (medication and physical interventions) has not helped sufficiently. You have developed a constellation of troubling symptoms.

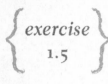

exercise
1.5

Pain Manifestations

Here is a list of some of the manifestations of chronic pain. Please check off those you have experienced.

_____ Feelings of depression, anger, worry, discouragement, and irritability.

_____ Sleep difficulties.

_____ Financial problems.

_____ Problems relating to others, causing significant disturbance in relationships.

_____ Inability to tolerate physical activities.

_____ Withdrawal from social activities.

_____ Inability to concentrate.

_____ Poor memory.

_____ Isolation from support systems, including family, friends, and coworkers.

_____ A decrease in sexual activity or performance.

_____ A decrease in self-esteem.

_____ Secondary physical problems.

_____ Problematic use of pain medications and/or alcohol or addiction.

_____ Avoiding work and leisure activities.

_____ Negative attitudes concerning everyday life.

_____ Other: _____

_____

Write about the feelings that come up as you review this list.

_____

_____

_____

_____

Many Have Difficulty Telling the Difference between Physical and Emotional Pain

If you identify with some of the features listed, your life is probably damaged significantly by chronic pain. Chances are your family has been gravely affected as well. Pain has invaded your life, and life has become drudgery. Depression can result and even lead to hopeless or suicidal feelings. The suffering that accompanies chronic pain (your emotional responses) is often *much greater* than the pain itself.

Furthermore, often your responses to the pain exacerbate the pain itself. You judge it (negatively of course), resist it, get angry at it, and try to get away from it, and *the pain gets worse*. In fact, much worse. Resisting the pain causes the pain to get worse.

Pain is not right or wrong, good or bad. Pain simply exists in your life.
You can change your experience of pain and your attitude toward it.

Developing a New Awareness _____

{ *exercise* 1.6 }

Let's try an experiment. Identify a source of pain in your body right at this moment. Get mad at it—tighten the muscles in the area—worry about how much worse it is getting—throw hatred and loathing right into the pain—feel the despair because this is the way it is and will always be. Hold these negative feelings for a few moments…

Now relax for a minute. Just take a deep, slow breath. If you are having any angry or despairing thoughts, try to set them aside for a moment. Just breathe. And breathe again. Try to loosen the muscles that you just tightened. Think about something positive—a memory, a favorite place, a song, a loved one. And relax. Keep breathing.

Write below about any emotions, thoughts, and spiritual or physical experiences that came up for you. Did you feel the pain get worse as you tightened your body and mind? Were you able to relax, and as you did, did the pain lessen? If not, what got in the way?

_____

_____

_____

_____

_____

_____

_____

_____

If you are caught in the negative spiral of chronic pain, it may seem like there is no way out, but that's not the truth. You now have some clues to your experience of pain and some potential ways out. As the simple exercise above demonstrates, when you tighten your muscles and send negative energy toward the pain, the pain gets worse. It's as straightforward as that. If you successfully reduced your muscle tension, stopped judging the experience as negative, and paid attention to your responses, the pain diminished, even if only a little. Always take notice of small improvements, for those add up. If you noticed your pain increase and then decrease with this exercise, you have just seen that *you have the beginning of the answer to chronic pain*. Please don't underestimate the significance of this!

A lot of the work you will be doing in this book will be to help you notice your pain, but notice it in a very different way. It will require that you be open to changing the experience, and you will be amazed at the differences in how your pain "feels."

These techniques cannot help but help—a little for some, a remarkable amount for others—and a lot depends on your openness, willingness, and tenacity in applying yourself to these ways of changing your thinking about your pain.

RECOMMENDED READING

A Day without Pain by Mel Pohl, MD, FASAM; Central Recovery Press.

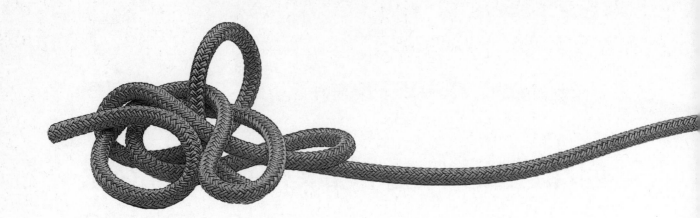

2

Chronic Pain and Addiction: Double Trouble

According to a 2006 study, 90 percent of all people in the US receiving treatment for pain management receive prescriptions for opioid medication. These medications carry with them a risk of dependency and addiction. For those with chronic pain who become addicted when they take opioids for pain relief, the two conditions exacerbate each other, making both worse than either would be alone. Many professionals believe the benefits of opioid treatment far outweigh the risk of developing addiction, but people who do become addicted find themselves in a conundrum: They need opioids to treat pain, but when they take them, they experience horrible consequences.

Given the complex and multifaceted nature of chronic pain and addiction, it is essential to address all the aspects of the condition—the physical, mental, emotional, and spiritual components—in order for the individual to recover. First, let's look at addiction in some detail.

Addiction Explained

Addiction is a complex brain disease. The symptoms of addiction include physical, emotional, spiritual, and thought disturbances with manifestations that affect behaviors and relationships. Use of drugs over time induces changes in the structure and function of the brain that can be long-lasting and produce a host of harmful effects. Studies have shown that in drug-addicted individuals, the areas of the brain that undergo physical changes are critical to judgment, decision making, emotion, memory, and behavior control. This may help explain the destructive behaviors of addiction. As the disease progresses, a person becomes increasingly unable to control his or her drug seeking and use even in the face of terrible consequences.

There is no way to predict with certainty whether a person will become addicted to drugs, but there are several known risk factors. These include:

- **Genes:** It is estimated that genetics accounts for 40 to 60 percent of a person's vulnerability to addiction.

- **Environment:** Frequent exposure to drug use in home, work, school, or social life can influence a person's use of drugs, which may become problematic.

- **Early use of drugs:** The earlier a person starts using drugs, the more likely he or she is to develop problems with abuse and addiction.

- **Mental illness:** Anxiety, depression, and other mood disorders are commonly associated with addiction.

- **Traumatic childhood experiences:** Abuse, neglect, dysfunction in the family, or other trauma can leave a child more susceptible to addiction later in life.

TERMINOLOGY OVERVIEW

Addiction is a chronic, relapsing brain disease characterized by compulsive drug seeking and use, despite harmful consequences. At one time, addiction was a pharmacologic term that referred to a person's using enough drugs to cause tolerance and physical dependence. In fact, we now know a person can have addiction without developing tolerance or physical dependence.

Tolerance means that more of the drug is needed over time to experience the same effect, and it commonly occurs with long-term use of opioids.

Physical dependence is characterized by being unable to stop using the drug without feeling terrible and developing a syndrome known as withdrawal.

Drug dependence is a synonym for addiction and is a set of behaviors involving problematic use of mood-altering substances over a continuous period of time. Symptoms a person might display include:

- Having problems with controlling use, and thus having an unpredictable outcome once he or she begins using a substance.

- Trying to cut down or stop, but being unable to "stay stopped."

- Being preoccupied with the drug and continuing to use it even though it is causing problems.

- Not doing the things he or she used to do and "chasing the high"—spending time and energy getting the drug and using it.

With addiction, the problem exists not so much with the drug itself, but with the way that drug works in the brain and nervous system. Some of you are destined to develop addiction because of how "well" the drug works—both physically and emotionally. You were probably wired differently from birth, and with continued exposure to a drug, particularly an opioid (whether you started taking it for pain or not), you eventually became addicted.

Some people develop tolerance and physical dependence. These phenomena occur with continued exposure to certain substances over time. With increased use of certain drugs (e.g., an opioid), the body reacts by decreasing the effect of the drug, in this case, pain relief. This is tolerance. Consequently, in order to achieve pain relief, you increase the dose of the drug. This adjustment works temporarily, but eventually the need for still-increased doses will occur. Eventually, the drug seems not to work any longer, which results in using stronger, more potent drugs in an escalating upward spiral.

If you become tolerant to the drug, this indicates that your body is "normalized" in the presence of the drug. In fact, you may become so used to the drug that you *need* the drug to feel normal. Without it, you feel terrible. This is physical dependence. When the drug is discontinued abruptly, you will feel withdrawal—in effect, the opposite feelings that the drug caused. So if opioids cause decreased pain and some amount of calm and well-being, then withdrawal consists of increased pain and anxiety, body aches, stomach and muscle cramps, diarrhea, nausea, vomiting, insomnia, and agitation. This outcome is one of the main reasons some of you will feel the need to continue the opioid, since, when you try to stop or even reduce the dose, you feel terrible.

So what is the solution to this awful problem? You feel that you have to take the drug to feel any level of pain relief, even though it barely works. In fact, as you'll learn, it actually may be making the pain worse due to a phenomenon known as opioid-induced hyperalgesia. You might consider cutting down the dose of the opioid; however, that presents the immediate problem of withdrawal. In the short run, cutting down or stopping will make you feel much worse. This is because the withdrawal of the opioid from your system inevitably causes a temporary increase in symptoms, including pain. This effect makes the process of coming off opioids challenging but not impossible. You may be tempted to substitute one opioid for another, which may temporarily delay the process.

We have treated hundreds of people with pain who are tolerant to and dependent on opioids. The withdrawal process is best done under medical supervision and temporarily, you are likely to feel worse. But on the other side, when the opioids have left your system for a week or two, your pain will diminish and you will start to feel better. The discomfort of withdrawal may continue for a while, even for several months in some, but eventually your nervous system will readjust to the absence of opioids and you will return to a state of well-being that has escaped you for years.

Addiction is a chronic disease similar to other chronic diseases such as type II diabetes, cancer, and cardiovascular disease.

–*National Institute on Drug Abuse*

Four Stages of Addiction

As with many illnesses, to understand the progressive nature of the disease of addiction, we have broken it down into stages. People who have addiction started in stage I and will inevitably end up in stage IV if not treated. The progression from stage I to IV may occur rapidly or may take years or decades. Stopping drug use might halt the disease process, but treatment is still necessary. Further, if use is restarted, the disease process will pick up where it left off. Like a passenger on a train traveling from New York to California, if you get off in Chicago (stage II), you will "reboard" in Chicago and continue west, heading inevitably toward stage IV, disability, and eventually death. Here are the stages in further detail:

STAGE I

Stage I addiction begins with the first ingestion of a mood-altering drug. The feelings that occur are related to mood change. This is often a sense of "normalizing" the world, euphoria, or an energized sense of well-being. This sensation may be especially true of the first use of opioid painkillers. The pain goes away—both the physical and the emotional pain. Although there may be no outward behavioral changes yet, such drug use cannot be considered "safe" because in persons with the neurobiological risk for developing addiction, subsequent use may result in substance abuse and life changes beyond the person's control.

At this stage, family members generally have a greater awareness of the problematic use of substances than the addict. The developing addict may have an uneasy sense that there is something wrong, but denies it to him- or herself and others. The addict in stage I may cut down or even quit using for periods of time, but without recovery or treatment, typically he or she eventually resumes use and the problems recur and escalate.

A person with chronic pain and addiction may be defensive about drug use and answer any criticism or questions about it by rationalizing, for example:

- **Explaining why drug use is necessary:** *I have to take these medicines for the pain so I can function,* or *The doctor said I need to take this.*

- **Minimizing the consequences of drug use:** *It's not that bad because I'm not taking that many,* or *I only take what's prescribed and sometimes less* (hoarding extras "just in case"), or *I go to work every day, so I can't have a problem.*

- **Denying:** *I don't have a problem with drugs.*

Other characteristics of stage I may include:

- Wanting the drug (craving).

- Counting pills.

- Worrying when the supply of pills is low.

- Focusing on the time until the next dose (preoccupation).

- Increasing the dose without a doctor's order (tolerance).

- Taking a pill or two in the morning to "get going" (using for purposes other than those intended by the prescriber).

- Adding another substance to supplement the effects (commonly alcohol or other sedatives).

- Using stimulants because of fatigue caused by the opioids.

This stage usually occurs in individuals who haven't had chronic pain for very long but are beginning to develop problems with opioids.

STAGE II

In stage II, the addict begins to experience the negative consequences of drug use. This stage is characterized by problems in one of the following major functional areas: family or home life, job or school function, social function, legal status, or health. In stage II you experience problems in one of these areas, although several areas may be affected as time goes on. Examples of stage II problems include:

- Fighting at home, neglecting familial responsibilities, or separation.

- Being disciplined at work or decreased work performance.

- Calling in sick frequently or missing work without calling.

- Failing a major test at school or dropping classes.

- Using illegal methods to obtain drugs (consulting other doctors but not disclosing this to each doctor, acquiring pills from illegal sources, using multiple doctors or pharmacies, driving under the influence), but not yet having been caught or arrested.

- Experiencing a worsening of health problems, many of which are side effects of opioids, such as escalating pain, nausea, constipation, diarrhea, headaches, sleep disturbance, fatigue, or depression.

This stage usually occurs in individuals who have been dealing with chronic pain for some time, and though they may appear okay on the outside, they are beginning to experience deterioration of function.

STAGE III

In this stage, there is intense preoccupation with the desire to experience mood-changing effects of the drug(s). Daily drug use, depression, and thoughts of suicide are common. Family troubles increase. Legal problems may ensue. Stage III is characterized by any one of the following major consequences in any one major functional area. If family function is the problem area, these consequences include:

- Being asked to move out for good, leading to the end of the relationship.

- Getting a divorce.

- Becoming estranged from close family members.

If the problem areas are outside the home, they could include any of the following:

- Getting fired.

- Failing out of school.

- Going to jail.

Stage III physical changes include:

- Being hospitalized.

- Being physically dependent on drugs; suffering withdrawal when trying to cut down or stop.

Again, for it to be considered stage III, the addict must have only one of these problems, not multiple problems in all areas of his or her life, even though that may be the case. This stage usually occurs in individuals who have been dealing with chronic pain for years and the amount and variety of their medications has steadily increased, with progressive decrease in function, dependence on the drug(s), and general worsening of quality of life.

STAGE IV

Stage IV is considered late-stage addiction, where the effects of the disease have spread to all areas of the person's life. Stage IV addiction, like stage IV cancer, is the period that precedes death from the disease. The length of time people can survive in this stage varies, but if the disease is treated, even at this point, the destructive process stops, life expectancy increases, and quality of life improves. Common causes of death from addiction include overdose, liver failure, accidents, suicide, and infections that would be preventable or treatable in nonaddicts. Those who have reached this stage need increasing quantities of drugs just to feel normal. Physical signs, such as damage to the heart, liver, and brain; malnutrition; lower resistance to pneumonia or tuberculosis; and overdoses are common.

Stage IV addiction is characterized by multiple problems in more than one major life area. Generally it means the person has no meaningful family life or relationships left, has no job or school life, is cognitively impaired by drug use, and has severe long-term, often permanent health consequences, including brain dysfunction. In stage IV, pain and addiction are deeply entrenched in a person's life and the person is alienated from loved ones and medical professionals alike. People with stage IV addiction fit the stereotype of those with addiction and are commonly homeless, in jail, or in an institution.

Individuals with chronic pain often have histories of overdosing on drugs, either accidentally or on purpose. The acetaminophen in their opioid medications has caused liver damage. Their lives consist of unending pain, periods of sleeping and sleeplessness, staying in bed most of the time, and trips to the emergency room, either to try to get drugs or for treatment of complications of the advanced disease.

Hopefully by now, you are beginning to understand addiction more clearly. In the next chapter, we will invite you to look at your use of substances and try to make sense of how these substances have affected your pain and your behavior. So open your mind and your heart and get ready to find some answers.

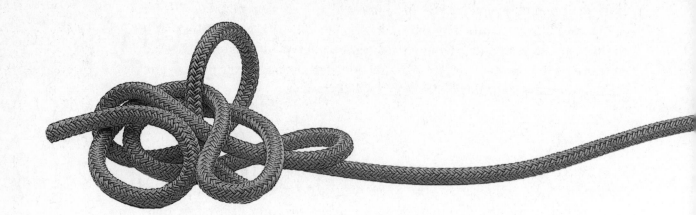

3

Am I an Addict?

Now that we have explained addiction, we would like to help you answer this question. We'll explore, in some depth, the reluctance, perhaps even overwhelming fear, that many with chronic pain have about addiction and the term "addict." If you don't consider the possibility that you have addiction, you may miss the opportunity to get better. In this chapter, we will not tell you whether or not you are an addict, but we will provide you with facts so that you can make an accurate and informed assessment.

The Stigma of Addiction

Why are the words "addiction" and "addict" so problematic for so many people? Much of this difficulty can be attributed to the stigma that is assigned to them. *Merriam-Webster's Collegiate Dictionary* defines stigma as "a mark of shame or discredit."* It is often attached to social judgment and cultural norms. The stigma attached to "addiction" and "addict" makes them "dirty" words. Despite volumes of research on drug dependence and scientific evidence to the contrary, addiction is viewed by many as a moral failing or weakness. Addicts and their families are subjected to social, legal, and financial discrimination, making it difficult for them to obtain the help they need. When addicts do access help, insurance is inadequate to cover the cost of effective treatment. Family members are often the most judgmental because they have experienced the consequences of the addict's behavior, not realizing the addict is sick, not "bad."

By permission. From Merriam-Webster's Collegiate® Dictionary, 11th Edition, ©2008 by Merriam-Webster, Incorporated (www.Merriam-Webster.com).

Addiction is one of the few diseases that carries such a negative emotional charge and is a source of shame or embarrassment. Who would want to have a diagnosis or label that carries such a stigma? For those with chronic pain who take opioids, attempting to discuss this topic is often met with resistance and denial.

{ *exercise* 3.1 }

Your View of Addiction _____

When you hear the word "addiction" or "addict," what is your emotional response?

_____

_____

_____

_____

_____

Do you believe either of these terms (addict, addiction) applies to you?
Why or why not?

_____

_____

_____

_____

_____

Addiction is a term that often conjures up negative stereotypes. You may relate to some and not to others. Write your stereotypes about addiction. Where do these ideas come from?

_____

_____

_____

_____

_____

I AM AN ADDICT

For some of you, there will be no question as to whether or not you are an addict—you already know you are. If you have experienced recovery you already understand it is extremely dangerous to put opioid painkillers in your system because eventually you will likely lose control and relapse, either with opioids or with other mood-altering drugs. For you, the main issue will be coming to terms with the fact that you can't safely take opioids for your chronic pain. You will need to find alternative treatments if you are to stay clean (drug-free) and in recovery. This also pertains to you if you identify as having other manifestations of addiction (e.g., alcohol, stimulants, sedatives, etc.), since the use of opioids will cloud your thinking and make it that much easier to compulsively drink, take drugs, gamble, overeat, and so on.

Pain recovery will work for you by complementing the program you are already working with your sponsor and by helping you realize that you can live with a certain amount of pain without taking medication.

For those of you who know or suspect you are an addict, but have never experienced recovery, this book can serve as your entry point to beginning a program and changing your life. By working a program and implementing the concepts of pain recovery, you can live without drugs and in recovery from both addiction and chronic pain.

Whether you know you have addiction, are unsure, or are convinced you are not an addict, we recommend you read this chapter. We feel strongly that the information it contains is essential to the process of pain recovery no matter what your circumstances.

FRED'S STORY

At thirty-six years old, I was in great shape. I had been clean and in recovery for twenty-six months. I was diligently working my recovery program with my sponsor. I stayed physically fit working as a furniture mover. For the first time in my life, I knew and accepted who I was. I had fully accepted that I was an addict and was reaping the benefits recovery had to offer.

One day at work, I was lifting a heavy piece of furniture and I felt something pop in my back. This began an ongoing nightmare of medical appointments and surgeries. Over the next three years, I went from being physically active and fit to not even being able to pick up or play with my stepchildren. Getting out of bed was a chore, sitting too long hurt, standing too long hurt, and in essence, doing anything hurt. My life was changed dramatically.

Even when the pain was tolerable, it was like having a constant toothache. I had to practice the principles of my program daily so I wouldn't act out in frustration, anger, and intolerance. Being inactive and unable to work resulted in weight gain and loss of self-esteem. Finances became an issue, and all this placed a tremendous strain on my relationships. I struggled not to play the role of victim even though my addiction told me I was a victim.

Then there was the issue of taking pain medication, which went against my basic belief in total abstinence. Part of me wanted to take something to relieve the pain, but I didn't because I was terrified of relapsing.

For at least a year I waited for each medical appointment and test, hoping there would be answers and a solution to my pain. The first doctor I went to said I pulled a muscle. The next doctor said it was probably my sciatic nerve, and stretched me on a machine that to me looked similar to torture racks used in medieval times. After several MRIs, X-rays, and injection of dyes into my back, the final diagnosis was three severely ruptured discs. I had minor surgery followed by months of rehabilitation, but the problem only got worse.

The decision to undergo major surgery had been a difficult process, but I could not go on living in pain every day. The surgery involved the insertion of six-inch pins and plates in my back. After that, I was given morphine while in the hospital. This was as traumatic for me as the surgery. I had so much fear that once I used, I would relapse. This was despite the fact that my sponsor, the doctor, and my support group told me it wasn't using; it was what I needed to heal. I prayed every night in the hospital, and my friends brought twelve-step meetings to me every day. I stopped taking morphine two days before I was released. Then the doctor told me I needed pain medication when I went home. Thanks to the advice of someone with a lot of clean time and experience, I filled only one prescription and never took more than I was supposed to. I called him every day to let him know how I was feeling and what I was taking. I was very aware of my addiction during this period because I was constantly focused on what time it was and when I needed to take the next pill. I wrote a list of pros and cons, did medication research, and ended up using only ibuprofen and a nonsteroidal anti-inflammatory drug when needed.

This experience taught me just how strong my addiction is, and that without the recovery support and experience, I would never have stayed clean. The support of my sponsor and friends kept me focused and helped me stay in the recovery process because I was, and always will be, an addict, whether I am in pain or not.

Is It Really about Choice?

Many view addicts' use of substances and related behaviors as a choice. People who have addiction may have made a decision at one time to use a drug, but they never made a decision to become addicted. The addict's brain was different before the first use of a drug, and scientific evidence has shown many of the significant ways the brain changes in response to chronic exposure to mood-altering drugs. According to Alan I. Leshner, Ph.D., former director of the National Institute on Drug Abuse (NIDA), "the evidence suggests that those long-lasting brain changes are responsible for the distortions of cognitive and emotional functioning that characterize addicts, particularly the compulsion to use drugs that is the essence of addiction."

Even if you never used a substance in the past and only started taking medication for your chronic pain, you may develop addiction. Just as an addict who uses for the first time is not choosing to become addicted, an individual with chronic pain who takes his or her first prescription would never choose and never intend to become addicted.

For those of you who are resistant to exploring the possibility that you are addicted, the issue may be getting past the stigma of addiction and letting go of the need to be better than an addict. Addiction is a no-fault illness, just like chronic pain.

At this point we don't want you to get stuck on whether or not you have addiction, but rather to focus on solutions to your problems. If you spend your energy trying to prove you are not an addict, you will limit the benefits you may receive from this book. We are not interested in labeling you. We are committed to helping you. You will decide for yourself in the long run.

If you are unsure at this point, we suggest you try a perspective such as "I am not sure if I am an addict or not, but I will have a clearer picture if I do the exercises and complete this book," or "Even if I decide I am not an addict, the solutions to addiction and chronic pain are so similar that I will benefit from this process and from applying what I learn to my life," or even "I think this is crazy, but I admit my way hasn't worked so far, so what do I have to lose?" For right now, try to suspend judgments and do the work. The closer you get to balance, the clearer things will become.

> There is no more shame in being an addict than there is in having chronic pain.

Arguments against Being an Addict

We realize at this point your head might still be saying, "But I'm not an addict. What are they talking about? I only used drugs as prescribed by my doctor." Frankly, it doesn't really matter. Or you may think, "I would never have developed problems with the drugs if I didn't have the pain." Again, it doesn't matter. As we have said, we aren't concerned with labels, and we also aren't concerned with your motivation or specific circumstances. We only care about what is happening in your life as a result of drug use and what you want to do about your situation. How you identify yourself—as addicted, drug-dependent, having problematic drug use, or simply a victim of circumstances—only matters if it prevents you from getting better.

The purpose of this book is to help you discover solutions that work no matter which label you most identify with. To say "I am an addict" is a personal decision that only you can make. However, to effectively determine the truth will require work on your part. Denying that you are an addict without examining the possibility that you are will prevent you from growing and finding balance. The following exercise deals with some of the ways people deny the possibility that they have addiction.

{ *exercise* }
3.2

I'm Not an Addict Because… _____

____ I have a problem with medications but I have to take them for my chronic pain.

____ I use prescribed medication and not illegal drugs.

____ I don't lie, cheat, steal, or live on skid row.

____ I've never snorted, smoked, or injected my pain medication.

If you have used any of the above statements, place a check next to it. If you are undecided or don't believe you are an addict, write your reasons here:

_____

_____

_____

_____

PAIN IN RECOVERY SUPPORT GROUP (PIRSG)

The Pain in Recovery Support Group (PIRSG) was created to provide those already in a twelve-step fellowship with a safe place to discuss their chronic pain issues in a mutually-supportive environment. For those not already in a twelve-step fellowship and who are seeking an opioid-free solution to their pain, PIRSG provides a place to practice the principles of pain recovery. PIRSG also offers information on various twelve-step fellowships so people can decide which one best fits their needs.

For more information about the PIRSG, please email info@forrecovery.org or visit www.paininrecovery.org.

Below you will find a self-test provided by the Pain in Recovery Support Group (PIRSG). The purpose of this exercise is to assess your use of medication and the possibility of addiction. We suggest you tear it off and make copies, and after you complete the self-test, ask family or friends to complete it also, with regard to your use. Getting input from others can expand your view of what your use has been like. When we are too close to a situation, those who care for us may provide perspective. If you feel resistant to doing this, just acknowledge the resistance and do it anyway. Don't prejudge what others may say; just get their input. Input is necessary to accurately assess and diagnose, and as with any medical condition, you need an accurate assessment and diagnosis to effectively deal with your problems. So stay open-minded and get as much information about your situation as you can. If you feel the information is inaccurate, be sure to discuss this at a later time with a trusted person, a counselor, or a professional.

Am I Addicted to My Pain Medication? Self-Test _____

{ *exercise* 3.3 }

The following questions may help you make that determination. Answer yes or no for each question.

_____ 1. Have you ever taken more of your medications or taken them more frequently than was prescribed?

_____ 2. Have you ever used another doctor because your doctor wouldn't prescribe any more medication or increase your dosage?

_____ 3. Do you find yourself looking at the clock to find out when you can take your medication next?

_____ 4. Have you used alcohol while taking prescriptions to enhance the medications' effect, even knowing you were not supposed to?

_____ 5. Have you ever used illegal drugs while taking prescribed medications?

_____ 6. Do you have more than one doctor who is prescribing medications for you?

   If yes, are those doctors aware of all of the medications you are taking?

_____ 7. Have you ever gone to an emergency room to get additional medications because the ones you had were not enough?

_____ 8. Have you ever run out of a prescription before you were supposed to because you used more than was prescribed?

_____ 9. Did you ever think "as needed" meant you could use as much as you wanted to, when you wanted to?

_____ 10. Have you ever lied to a doctor about why you needed another prescription filled?

_____ 11. Have you ever exaggerated your reported pain level just in case you had more pain later or to get another or a stronger prescription?

_____ 12. Did you have addiction problems before your chronic pain?

_____ 13. Have you ever thought, "I can't live without medication"?

_____ 14. Have you ever gotten a prescription and lied to your spouse or other family or friends about it?

_____ 15. Have you ever lied to your spouse or mate or anyone about how much medication you are taking?

_____ 16. Are you taking prescription medication and supplementing it with over-the-counter medication?

_____ 17. Are you taking other prescriptions to deal with the side effects of your pain medication, e.g., sleep aids, stimulants, antianxiety drugs, or Soma?

_____ 18. Have you ever taken anyone else's pain medication?

_____ 19. Have you ever stolen, forged, or altered a prescription, or called in a prescription by impersonating medical staff?

_____ 20. Have you ever crushed, snorted, or injected your medication or taken it in a way other than the way it was intended to be taken?

_____ 21. Have you ever overdosed or needed medical help because you took too much medication?

_____ 22. Have you ever experienced a blackout (memory loss) caused by medication?

_____ 23. Have you experienced legal consequences as a result of taking your medication, such as a DUI or assault and battery arrest?

_____ 24. Have you had a friend, spouse, or family member express concern regarding your use of pain medication?

_____ 25. Have you ever taken pain medications to deal with other issues such as stress or anxiety?

None of these questions necessarily defines addiction, but if you answered "yes" to any of these, you should not rule out the possibility of addiction. The more "yes" answers you have, the greater the cause for concern about addiction. Do not use this test to judge yourself negatively; use it as part of a process of learning and examining that is necessary for success in pain recovery.

Problematic Drug Use (PDU)

For many of you with chronic pain, addiction may be too much of a stretch. However, you may find it helpful to look at your use of medications as being either problematic or nonproblematic. Even before a diagnosis of addiction is established, you may conclude there is problematic use that may or may not evolve into addiction. The following table will assist you in defining problematic use.

Nonproblematic Prescription Drug Use	Problematic Prescription Drug Use
Pain is relieved or manageable with medications.	No appreciable decrease in pain.
No significant changes in functioning due to medication.	Significant decrease in functioning due to medication.
No significant effect on relationships; no concerns from family regarding use.	Ongoing relationship problems and concerns from family regarding use.
Able to work with no significant decrease in job performance.	Unable to work or significant impairment due to medication.
Stable or maintenance dose of pain medication.	Steadily increasing dose and frequency of medications with little or no decrease in pain.
Emotional stability and acceptance of any physical limitations.	Emotional instability and increasing lack of acceptance regarding physical limitations.
No significant cognitive impairment due to medication use.	Significant cognitive impairment due to use e.g., foggy thinking, difficulty concentrating, memory problems.
Using medications only for pain relief.	Relying on medications for emotional effect.

{ *exercise* }
3·4

Use of Medications _____

Write about areas in your life related to the previous chart where you are experiencing problems.

_____

_____

_____

_____

_____

_____

If you are experiencing PDU, what do you propose to do about it?

_____

_____

_____

_____

Usually people begin taking medication to manage physical pain, but at some point, often without realizing it, start using the medication to manage emotional pain as well. Eventually the medications no longer work for long or very well to ease the physical or emotional pain, and the side effects may actually cause more physical and emotional pain. This happens because long-term use of opioids can increase the body's and brain's pain signals. This is called pain rebound syndrome or opioid-induced hyperalgesia. In the end, medication use that started as a reasonable treatment approach to relieve suffering can be the cause of problems in all areas of your life.

From this point on, we will use the terms "addiction" and "problematic drug use" or "PDU" interchangeably. Use the term that feels right to you, keeping in mind that regardless of how you choose to label your situation, the principles of pain recovery apply.

Pain and PDU: Four Stories

1. JR had a history of alcohol abuse—twelve to twenty-four beers per day, shots on weekends, blackouts, and a DUI fifteen years ago. He also smoked and snorted one to two grams of cocaine per day for a few years. After his DUI, the court ordered him to attend twelve-step meetings. Much to his surprise, he attended, grew to like the meetings, got a sponsor, and worked the Twelve Steps. His recovery was going well—so well that he got married, got promoted, and was so busy with family and work that he stopped going to meetings. Six months later, he lifted a heavy box in his garage and sprained his back. An MRI showed no significant cause for his pain, and his doctor started him on Lortab and Soma, with Ambien to help him sleep. Before he realized it, he was taking the entire thirty-day prescription in the first nine days, and for the rest of the month he would beg and borrow more drugs, eventually resorting to stealing drugs from his ailing mother or buying them on the street. He would drink when he ran out of pills, which became a more frequent occurrence. Clearly, he had reactivated his addiction and required treatment, which got him reengaged in the recovery process. He also needed to acquire tools to deal with his pain without medications. He admitted that he had been taking the pills for all sorts of reasons, including to relax, to get energy, and sometimes just to get high.

2. Deirdre wonders how this happened to her. She was a regular working stiff, living in a nice house with her husband and two kids. She never used drugs to any great extent; she didn't like them. She had tried cocaine and pot when she was younger and got drunk on weekends in college but that's about it. She had hardly had more than a glass of wine with dinner once a month for the past few years. She lost her taste for alcohol when she started taking pain pills. Her mom was a pill addict, and she never wanted to be like her. Then she developed pelvic pain and adhesions after surgery for endometriosis. She found that one or two Lortab in the morning took the pain away and got her going better than a double espresso. So she started using the pills to get going, keep going, and relieve the pain. When the doctor gave her Soma, she could calm down, numb out, and sleep—she was hooked. The pain was a great excuse, and her doctors were perfect accomplices. She progressed from Lortab to Percocet, which she was getting from her pain doctor, internist, GI doctor, and gynecologist, and neither she nor they realized what was happening. She eventually found that chewing the pills gave her a more intense high. A few months ago she started buying from friends, and now she is spending $500 a month on pills. She's up to twenty pills a day. She knows she is out of control, addicted, and needs help, but she's mystified—how did this happen to her? After all, it just started with the pain! She's not even sure if she's in pain or not anymore.

3. May wants off medications, but feels she is not an addict. She never abused drugs, took anyone else's prescription, or stole to support herself. Her medications are all prescribed by her doctor. She wants to try going off meds because they have significant side effects—she is not herself. She sleeps a lot and her pain is still pretty bad. The medications don't work as well as they used to, and she's taking stronger medications in higher doses. She heard that stopping meds may decrease her pain, although she finds that hard to believe. She developed fibromyalgia ten years ago and has no life. Her husband left and her grown kids don't come around, and she doesn't blame them. She sleeps most of the time, and when she's awake she's depressed, grumpy, and complaining. And the constipation is killing her! She thinks of an addict as someone who lives on the street. Addicts take medications to get high. They lie, cheat, and steal. She doesn't do those things. Her dad was an alcoholic and she doesn't ever want to act the way he did. He was abusive and downright hateful. She never drank because of that, and tried pot only a few times as a kid. She takes no other drugs except what is prescribed. She doesn't buy that she's an addict and doesn't want to participate in addiction treatment, but she wants off the medications and doesn't know how she'll be able to live with the pain. She is consumed with fear all the time. She's angry at herself for not being stronger, at her husband for leaving, and at the doctors for allowing this to happen.

4. Henry doesn't think he has addiction and doesn't want off his drugs, but THEY want him to stop. He sustained a fracture of his lumbar spine and herniated three discs in 2001. He hasn't worked since. He is angry at the person who left the floor wet and slippery, which caused him to slip and fall. He is furious with the workers' comp company and especially with the case manager who wouldn't let him have another surgery and who delayed his MRI. They generally made his life miserable. He is angry at his wife for any number of reasons and irritable with his kids. They can barely get by on the money he gets from disability, and as for his lawyer, the SOB won't even call him back. He is miserable and depressed. He is in a dead-end life that on many days he wishes would end. On Tuesday he was confronted by all of them—wife, lawyer, case manager, doctor; even his poor kids were dragged into it. He couldn't stand the tears, and in fact, he can't stand emotion at all. So he agreed to detox and try to stay off medications and do something different with his pain. On a scale of one to ten, his optimism about success was a zero, but at least he'd get them all off his back. He can't imagine living without his medications. How will he sleep? he wonders (even though he never sleeps now for more than an hour or two). Medications were the only thing that made his life tolerable—that and lying perfectly still until the meds kicked in and he was able to fall asleep. Not much of a life, but what else was there? He was adjusted to this life, such as it was, and now THEY want to mess it up.

Pain and PDU: Which Type Are You? _____

Did you relate to any of these stories? Write which you most related to and why.

_____

_____

_____

_____

_____

The examples of these individuals illustrate the four types of clients seeking help for chronic pain whom we generally find in the Chronic Pain Rehabilitation Program at LVRC:

1. You identify as having addiction. You know you are an addict and have experienced recovery. Due to chronic pain issues, you have relapsed in an attempt to relieve or control your pain.

2. You had no history of addiction, but you started on pain medications and now you are out of control. You are addicted and unable to stop or regain control of your life, and you are beginning to realize this and what you have to do—that is, stop the drugs.

3. You do not believe that you are an addict. You take only the medications prescribed by your doctor, *but* your life is not better with pain-relieving drugs; in fact, it's worse. Even though you are taking medications, your pain is increasing rather than being controlled. Your dosage is escalating in the face of inadequate pain relief, and your function is more impaired since you've been on the drugs. You're reluctant to do anything lest it make the pain worse.

4. You in no way think you have a problem with your medications or addiction, but someone else does. This may be a spouse, significant other, parent or child, employer, doctor, counselor, therapist, lawyer, judge, workers' compensation company, or others in your life. This person or organization is *making* you do something about your drug use. (Does anyone or anything really *make* you do something?) You're in pain and you don't think it can get any better. You are convinced that coming off medication will make your pain and your life worse. You may even think you need more medication, not less.

Write about which of these four types best describes your understanding of your condition and how you feel about it. These categories are not mutually exclusive. You may feel one fits you best, you may relate to several, or you may not be sure which best describes you.

_____

_____

_____

_____

_____

Am I Addicted? Here's Why It Matters

If you have addiction (type one or type two), you have a "loss-of-control" disease. No addict regains control over mood-altering drugs, so the only safe treatment is abstinence. Since you have chronic pain, opioids are likely to be prescribed, and as you can see, *any* use of opioids, even though prescribed, can trigger this loss-of-control phenomenon. What a dilemma—you are really between a rock and a hard place. You can't keep going as you are because the drugs are too destructive in your life, but you can't picture your life without the medications and wonder how you will manage your pain without them. It seems like a no-win situation.

If you don't see yourself as addicted (type three or type four), then you have a more challenging task of deciding how to proceed. We have found that if opioids are causing problems (side effects, increased pain, and decreased function), the *safest* course for you is to discontinue the opioids completely. It is a logical next step to stop medications if you are having problems with them and they are ultimately making your life worse, are not helping your pain, and might even be causing *more* pain. Labeling this as addiction may or may not be helpful at this time.

If someone is pressuring you to do something about your drug use, we strongly encourage you to ask yourself why. Try not to get drawn into defending the drug use; try to put yourself in their shoes and understand why that person or entity is suggesting you have PDU.

*Revisiting the Stages of Addiction*_____

{ exercise 3.6 }

Review the stages of addiction presented in Chapter Two on pages 20-23. Does one stage best describe your situation? You may find you have characteristics of more than one stage.

_____

Why did you pick this stage? If you chose more than one stage, explain.

_____

_____

_____

_____

Regardless of which stage(s) you identify with, the basic solution is the same, and treatment works. But the earlier, the better. As with any chronic disease, better treatment options exist before the disease has spread to all parts of the body. If your disease has progressed, which is often the case if you have chronic pain and addiction, you may end up needing more-involved and longer-term treatment. It is best to consult with a professional who is familiar with co-occurring chronic pain and addiction.

Finding Recovery

In order to stay clean, balanced, and in recovery, obsessive thoughts (mental), compulsive use (physical), avoidance of feelings (emotional), and self-centered behavior (spiritual) need to be addressed. Not dealing with these aspects results in relapse. The same applies to problematic use of prescription drugs for chronic pain.

Recovery Is More than Abstinence from Drugs _____

{ exercise 3.7 }

Addiction is a mental obsession, causing overpowering thoughts about using despite the problems it causes. Write about obsessive thoughts regarding your use of prescription drugs.

_____

_____

_____

_____

Addiction is a physical compulsion, causing loss of control over using. Write about your compulsive behaviors regarding prescription drugs.

_____

_____

_____

_____

Addiction is an emotional disorder, resulting in avoidance of feelings. Write about feelings you are avoiding with your use of prescription drugs for chronic pain.

_____

_____

_____

_____

Addiction is a spiritual disease, manifesting in self-centered behavior. Write about self-centered behaviors you have acted out with because of prescription drug use for chronic pain.

_____

_____

_____

_____

Moving Forward

We want to be clear that the process of recovery is the same whether your substance use has been entirely related to your chronic pain diagnosis or it started before your chronic pain. For you to get better, it does not matter whether your use was entirely medically-managed or you got your drugs from the Internet or a dealer. In many ways, _how_ your problems came to exist in your life is of minimal importance unless knowing this information helps you learn how to change your life for the better. The past is not unimportant, but you can start by knowing what the issues are in this moment and then move forward from there.

Often, people with chronic pain and addiction spend time and energy trying to figure out who is to blame for what has happened. We find that it is not helpful to assign blame. It is much more effective to stay focused on discovering and implementing solutions.

Use the label or labels that you feel comfortable with for now. Work on the exercises and expand your knowledge and insight. At some point you will probably come to a determination or a deeper understanding of what feels true, but for now this is not necessary. Let's move along to look at pain recovery, which encompasses the solutions we have been talking about. We believe it will work for you.

WEB RESOURCES

National Institute on Drug Abuse (NIDA): www.nida.nih.gov

Substance Abuse and Mental Health Services Administration (SAMHSA): www.samhsa.gov

RECOMMENDED READING

Narcotics Anonymous, Sixth Edition; Narcotics Anonymous World Services, Inc.

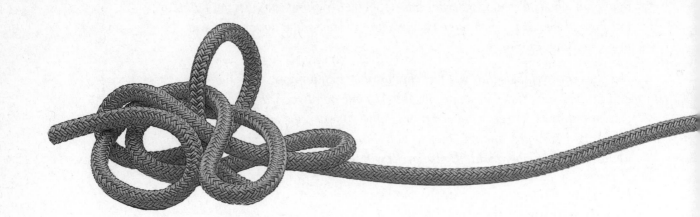

4

What Is Pain Recovery?
Changing Your Experience of Pain

Many who seek help for chronic pain are lost and confused, and aware of no option other than taking opioid medications as part of traditional treatment. Yet medication-based pain management often does not work, and regular use of opioids is a problem in and of itself. If traditional pain management has not worked for you, there is an alternative solution. Pain recovery is a comprehensive, opioid-free approach that entails safely discontinuing pain medication, decreasing the level of existing physical pain, and reducing mental, emotional, and spiritual suffering.

Our concept of pain recovery was developed after looking at how individuals with chronic pain could be helped by an approach similar to the recovery process for people with addiction. Recovery leads addicts to a new way of life through a process that includes abstaining from mood-altering drugs; addressing the physical, mental, emotional, and spiritual aspects of their disease; building mutual support and allies; and taking positive action.

In our observations of addicts who are successful in recovery and of individuals with chronic pain who are off pain medication and living a fulfilled life, we found many similarities. The qualities that recovering addicts have developed allow them to find a better way to live and even feel grateful for their chronic disease, not unlike others who face and transcend adversity—people we admire, who motivate us and seem to "rise above" or deal with life's problems in an effective and healthy manner. These kinds of people live lives that exemplify what we strive for in pain recovery and how we can change our experience of chronic pain from a negative to a positive.

Similarities between Chronic Pain and Addiction

Characteristics	Chronic Pain	Addiction
EPIDEMIOLOGY		
An estimated one in three Americans	✓	
An estimated one in four Americans		✓
DISEASE COURSE		
Chronic, progressive, intermittent worsening of symptoms, debilitating, can be fatal if untreated	✓	✓
HUMAN COST		
Suffering; decrease in functional ability; harm to self, family, community	✓	✓
FINANCIAL COST		
Over one hundred billion dollars per year and increasing	✓	✓
TREATMENT LENGTH		
Lifelong	✓	✓
PROGNOSIS		
Affected people and health care providers treating them are powerless over chronic pain/addiction, but neither individuals nor providers are helpless	✓	✓
TREATMENT/RECOVERY		
• Abstinence from mood-altering substances	✓	✓
• A program of recovery	✓	✓
• Challenging old and implementing new beliefs and thought patterns	✓	✓
• Acquiring and applying coping skills	✓	✓
• Addressing imbalances in the physical, mental, emotional, and spiritual self	✓	✓
• Developing healthy relationships	✓	✓
• Taking positive action	✓	✓
FAMILY ISSUES		
• Codependency	✓	✓
• Rebuilding lost trust	✓	✓
• Unhealthy boundaries	✓	✓

Pain Is Inevitable

Pain is a part of life and cannot successfully be
now you are left with what to do with your pain.
multidimensional—it's much more than your bo
stinging, burning, or whatever other sensations pl
(emotional), feeling alone or unsupported (spiritu
every day (mental). If your goal is to eliminate all ρ
will be painkilling drugs such as opioids. Even with
may not be gone, and the use of opioids will create i
emotional, mental, and spiritual self (suffering).

The question remains: What to do about pain? While
suffering is modifiable. Once you understand and acce
how to deal with the inevitable painful issues and condi
are essentially two paths you can take. Neither can elimi
to healing and personal growth while the other leads to o

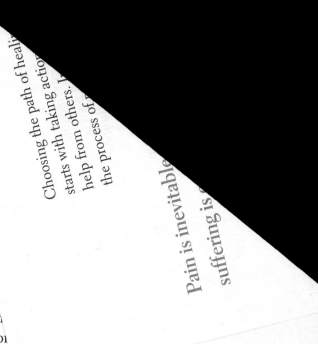

Choosing the path of heali
starts with taking actio
help from others.
the process of

Pain is inevitable
suffering is

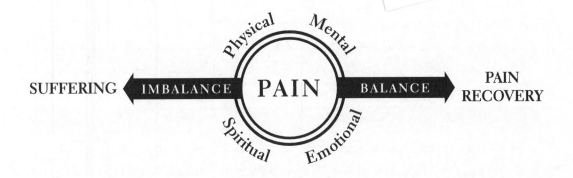

SUFFERING   IMBALANCE   **PAIN**   BALANCE   **PAIN RECOVERY**

Physical — Mental — Spiritual — Emotional

You choose the path of suffering when you attempt to eliminate all pain by avoiding,
masking, and medicating. This approach does not eliminate all pain and results in
imbalance in other areas of your life. The more you attempt to avoid, mask, and
medicate, the greater your suffering will be.

Choosing the path to pain recovery means you must give up the quest for "no more
pain." Rather, you begin by acknowledging and accepting your pain. Recovery starts
with recognizing that pain is an essential part of life and does not need to be feared or
avoided. By leaning into the pain, by simply allowing it to be there without resistance,
you become empowered to change the way you experience it. Rather than attempting
to eliminate your pain, you can change your goals to achieving manageable levels of
physical pain, increasing function, and reducing suffering. This is not being pain-free,
but this is pain recovery.

...ng and growth will require work on your part. The work
...n—completing exercises, sharing and accepting feedback and
...n order to do this, you will need to learn to trust and have faith in
...pain recovery.

optional and modifiable.

After years of battling her chronic pain by using powerful prescription painkillers, Deanna realized more medication wasn't the solution. In the following story, she describes how she was able to find a better way to live and how acceptance of her pain was an essential element in her recovery.

DEANNA'S STORY

The pain hit me one day right before my freshman year of college. I began to get terrible headaches every day and I couldn't do anything to make them stop. My head would pound so bad that I couldn't get out of bed, and I didn't want to be around anyone or near any loud noises. Anything that was stimulating was annoying, and all I wanted to do was sleep in a cool, dark room.

I went to see my primary care doctor looking for some answers, and, when nothing out of the ordinary came up, he sent me to a well-known neurologist and headache specialist in the area. I had what seemed like every test done to me, including MRIs, spinal taps, etc., and nothing was showing up. They tried putting me on almost every type of seizure medication, antidepressant, and mood stabilizer available, and I was still in a lot of pain. When everything seemed unbearable to me, the doctor offered me what seemed to be the only solution — narcotic pain medication. They didn't start out small with me. I remember getting tons of injectable morphine during an episode where my headache had lasted for more than five days.

As the year passed, my pain continued to increase and nothing was helping. Finally they put me on so much pain medication — "benzos" and different psychiatric drugs — that I had a major breakdown and entered psychiatric rehab. Taking these medications in the wrong doses and combinations and being in so much pain led me down a path to feeling like I wanted to die. I hated being in that much pain all the time! I truly believed there was something wrong with me and that I had nothing to live for. Although I did not get off all of the medications, I was able to clear my head of some of the mess and move to a lower dose of methadone.

At that time my headaches were not occurring daily, but they were still very much a distraction. I wanted to make it through college so I went on Duragesic for three years. Things weren't easy, but I didn't want that to get in the way of graduating. The medication kept the pain at bay, but I was never clear-headed. Sometimes I would still have to stay home. Nothing was ever perfect, and my head pounded the majority of the time.

After I made it through school, I decided to see if I could deal with my pain without the pain meds. I detoxed off the Duragesic and got a job in sales. I made it about a month, but didn't even know how to live my life without being on pain medication. I feared being in pain every day. Every time my head hurt I thought that I needed to have some sort of medication. I was afraid to be without something to take for my pain. Being in chronic pain felt like a death sentence—so unfair—and the problem seemed to have only one solution. I couldn't see an alternative, so I went back to the only thing I knew worked, which was pain pills. I went on OxyContin.

After I had been on "Oxys" and other painkillers for many years, my family helped me realize that opioid pain medication was not the answer to my chronic pain management. I went to treatment for ten weeks and learned different methods to deal with pain, along with other ways to think about my pain. Now I recognize it as something that is part of me and not something that I hate or a death sentence. I am one with my pain, and it is no longer "out to get me" or "against me." I recognize it and then I let it pass. I get massages, go to the chiropractor, use breathing exercises, and take safe, nonnarcotic pain medications recommended by an addiction specialist. I no longer see my pain as the evil force I did before. It might always be with me, but at least I can manage it today in ways that do not include pain medication and a hateful attitude.

Don't fight your pain; you can't win.
The paradox of recovery is that you have to surrender to win.
Accepting what you cannot change makes the difference.

Pain Isn't the Whole Problem, Nor Is the Absence of Pain the Whole Solution

If a miracle occurred and suddenly your pain was completely gone, everything would be fine, right? After all, isn't pain the problem? Actually, there is more to this picture: You would still need to deal with the damage caused to yourself and others because of the chronic pain. Even though you would no longer feel physical pain, you would probably still be in poor physical shape due to lack of exercise and unhealthy eating habits. Your thought processes would be the same, and the emotional and spiritual impact of living with pain for so long would remain. You might also still be dependent on medications and, in essence, have physical and emotional dependency on them. Unless you address your thoughts, feelings, spirit, relationships, and behaviors, the *only* thing that changes is your physical pain. Addressing the rest is the difference between absence of pain or abstinence from medication and pain recovery. Physical pain is only a small part of the big picture.

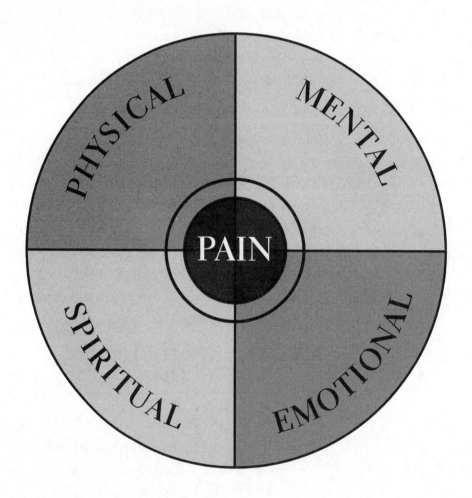

The following exercise is designed to give you a clearer picture of the total impact of chronic pain on your life and help you to understand why the absence of physical pain alone will not solve all your problems.

Causes of Imbalance _____ {exercise 4.1}

The following are issues that lead to imbalance in your life and contribute to your negative experience of pain. Check all that apply and add any that are not included.

PHYSICAL IMBALANCE

_____ 1. Lack of exercise

_____ 2. Poor eating habits

_____ 3. Loss of physical abilities

_____ 4. Loss of function

_____ 5. Insomnia or sleeping too much

_____ 6. Sexual problems

_____ 7. Inability to work and support yourself and your family

_____ 8. Other: _____

MENTAL IMBALANCE

_____ 1. Negative thoughts

_____ 2. Thinking you are a victim

_____ 3. Believing you have no control of your life

_____ 4. Thinking things are worse than they are

_____ 5. Other: _____

EMOTIONAL IMBALANCE

_____ 1. Depression

_____ 2. Guilt and shame

_____ 3. Anger and resentment

_____ 4. Unresolved childhood issues

_____ 5. Fear

_____ 6. Anxiety

_____ 7. Poor self-image

_____ 8. Other: _____

SPIRITUAL IMBALANCE

_____ 1. No sense of purpose in life

_____ 2. Lack of trust

_____ 3. Lack of faith

_____ 4. Feelings of isolation

_____ 5. Alienation from God/spirit/Higher Power

_____ 6. Other: _____

Four Points of Balance for Pain Recovery

The four points of balance are applicable to any situation in life, including chronic pain. In order for you to successfully practice pain recovery, you need to be off medications or working toward getting off of them. The next four chapters will go into detail on each point; for now, we will give a brief overview of balance in each of the four points. We will also ask you to identify patterns you learned early in life which may be affecting your current state of balance.

1. PHYSICAL BALANCE

Physical balance requires you to be mindful and respectful of your body, which includes paying attention to the messages it sends to your brain. You evaluate the state of your body thoroughly and continually, without becoming preoccupied. "How am I feeling? If there is pain, where is it coming from and how bad is it? What action that has worked in the past might I take to modify it—stretch, change position, get up and move, breathe, listen to soothing music, talk to someone (reach out), or share with someone who is hurting worse (give back)?"

With physical balance, you have an organized series of maintenance and crisis interventions. For example, a good maintenance regimen that keeps your pain tolerable consists of regular exercise, meditation, getting massages, stretching, and chiropractic, in addition to taking balancing actions we will describe in upcoming chapters.

Crisis intervention is used to counteract a painful flare-up. If you slept wrong and your back is really throbbing or you twisted your shoulder while lifting something heavy or it is raining and cold, causing your joints to ache—these can cause an acute worsening of your usual painful state and need to be addressed without medication for you to stay in balance.

Here are some common characteristics of a balanced physical experience:

- Eating nutritious foods.

- Avoiding toxins.

- Exercising regularly.

- Getting enough sleep.

- Practicing relaxation.

Physical Patterns

{ *exercise* 4.2 }

Many of our physical patterns were developed early in life. Write about some of the patterns you learned in your childhood that affect your physical condition today.

_____

_____

_____

_____

How might these patterns affect your chronic pain?

_____

_____

_____

_____

2. MENTAL BALANCE

With mental balance, you challenge the assumptions you have about your pain. Your pain is neither the worst that ever happened nor is it insignificant. It is not a punishment; it is simply an occurrence in the course of life that has various challenging ripple effects. Balanced thinking results in creating a realistic set of goals and focusing energy and effort into making progress toward achieving each one. This leads to improvement of pain, decreased suffering, and increased function, empowering you to set new goals and work toward achieving them. With mental balance, pain recovery is based not on blind faith but on well-thought-out, realistic expectations and progressive success achieved by applying the tools you learn from this book, and paying attention to this progress.

You actively and patiently change your thought patterns, knowing it happens neither easily nor quickly. However, your thoughts remain consistent in the belief that if you apply the techniques and practice the skills learned in pain recovery, your thinking will stay balanced. You understand that the most effective way to acquire new skills or, for that matter, to get better at anything, be it sports, cooking, auto repair, gardening, or pain recovery, is to:

1) Learn the techniques that work, and

2) Practice them relentlessly.

Here are some common characteristics of a balanced mental experience:

◉ Keeping a positive attitude.

◉ Paying attention to and challenging your thoughts.

◉ Setting achievable goals.

◉ Being open-minded and willing to try new things.

◉ Having realistic hope.

{ *exercise* 4·3 } *Mental Patterns* _____

Many of our thought patterns were developed early in life. Write about some of the patterns you learned in your childhood that affect your thinking today.

_____

_____

_____

_____

How might these patterns affect your chronic pain?

_____

_____

_____

_____

3. EMOTIONAL BALANCE

With emotional balance, you accept your emotions and know that it's okay to feel whatever you are feeling. You are more independent from the opinions and beliefs of others and pay closer attention to your inner voice. First, you need to identify your feelings and recognize that your feelings are a major part of you. Noticing and accepting your feelings is therefore a major part of self-acceptance. This does not mean you wish to stay as you are, but when you first see and accept who you are in the present moment, it allows you to make positive changes in your life. Accepting your feelings takes less energy than trying to deny or suppress them. Also, accepting your feelings sometimes helps prevent them from recurring over and over and enables you to change them. Finally, fully accepting your feelings allows you to shift your energy to productive thoughts or actions.

With emotional balance you feel your full emotional experience, recognizing that all feelings are part of you—you don't need to avoid any of them. You accept your feelings without labeling them good or bad, healthy or unhealthy.

You resolve old issues that you have avoided for one reason or another and work to heal and release your connection to the past, allowing yourself to be free to live in the moment. You are able to feel emotions for each circumstance that shows up in your life without troublesome attachment to old feelings.

Here are some common characteristics of a balanced emotional experience:

- Understanding feelings are neither good nor bad (not judging feelings).

- Seeing that simply experiencing emotions will not hurt you; in fact, *not* feeling emotions makes you hurt worse.

- Knowing that feeling results in healing, and avoidance results in ongoing suffering.

- Knowing that balanced thoughts create balanced emotions.

Emotional Patterns

Many of our emotional patterns were developed early in life. Write about some of the patterns you learned in your childhood that affect how you deal with or avoid feelings today.

_____

_____

_____

_____

How might these patterns affect your chronic pain?

_____

_____

_____

_____

4. SPIRITUAL BALANCE

With spiritual balance you are connected to the way you think and feel, and how you take care of your body. When balanced, your spirituality enhances your life. You do positive things that make you feel good, and you help others. You are in harmony with the world and those in it. Whatever life brings, you are able to deal with it and know you are okay. You are able to find meaning and purpose even in situations that are painful and not to your liking. You live in and accept each day as it comes, changing yourself instead of trying to change others.

Here are some common characteristics of a balanced spiritual experience:

- Accepting who you are and your place in the world.

- Having a sense of purpose and meaning.

- Being open to challenging your beliefs.

- Drawing on a source of inner and outer strength.

- Having values, beliefs, standards, and ethics that you embrace.

- Being aware and appreciative of a "transcendent dimension" to life beyond self.

- Having increased awareness of a connection with self, others, God/Spirit/Divine, and nature through regular spiritual practice.

Spiritual Patterns _____

Many of our spiritual patterns were developed early in life. Write about some of the patterns you learned in your childhood that affect your spirituality today.

_____

_____

_____

_____

How might these patterns affect your chronic pain?

_____

_____

_____

_____

CHRONIC PAIN AND TWELVE-STEP RECOVERY

What does chronic pain have to do with twelve-step recovery? A critical element of pain recovery is developing relationships within which you can build mutual support and allies. Twelve-step fellowships provide mutual support and allies to help you stay in pain recovery. Working the Twelve Steps is also an excellent way to assist you in finding balance. The underlying principles of the Twelve Steps work as well with our chronic pain clients as they do with addiction clients.

Going to meetings, getting a sponsor, and working the steps can help you learn how to effectively deal with the many aspects of chronic pain that contribute to suffering. No harm can come from such investigation, and you may be amazed at how helpful the fellowship and principles will be for you. Some of the key principles of the Twelve Steps are:

- Surrender.
- Honesty.
- Open-mindedness.
- Willingness.

Of course, for you to be successful in recovery you must be an active and willing participant in the process.

Relationships

You will recognize that the more balanced you are in the four points, the better your relationships will be. Achieving this improvement will take effort on your part, and again you will find yourself changing in relationship to others. You know that your health will cause you to attract other healthy people. You choose relationships that support and nurture you without being codependent or enabling. As a result of your healthy choices, you have individuals who lovingly tell you the truth because they put your well-being above their own fear. You ask for help whenever needed, knowing this is a sign of strength, not weakness.

You will attract others who have problems with chronic pain because they see the change in you and they are also interested in a solution. You freely share your solutions with them. You don't try to control them because you know everyone has to walk his or her own path, but you know you can provide guidance for them and share your own journey of experience, strength, and hope.

You evaluate all your relationships, looking at which ones drain you and which ones enhance your life. Knowing that drastic change will create imbalance, you create a plan to move toward building positive relationships and move away from negative relationships. You understand you will have fear, but you know you do not have to go through this alone.

Actions

As a result of continuous work to balance the four points, you are now able to face and adjust the manifestations of finding balance—your actions. Balanced actions include taking responsibility for yourself: showing up and participating in activities, getting out of bed, and taking care of your life.

You develop and execute healthy responses to troublesome thoughts and feelings. You take care of yourself by exercising, meditating, getting enough sleep, and eating properly. You work hard, arrive on time, participate in family activities, and refrain from gossip. Right action includes the "golden rule:" do unto others as you would have them do unto you. It also includes participating in support groups and giving to others as well as accepting help.

And finally, when your actions are balanced, you take the needed steps to deal with increased pain that may occur from time to time to ensure that you don't take opioids.

The Nature of Balance

Balance is not static but fluid, in a constant state of flux, much like the ebb and flow of the waves of the ocean. As the circumstances of your life change, so will your state of balance. Balance, then, is the journey, not the destination, and you are the navigator. No one else steers your ship, but people, circumstances, and events can create obstacles along the way. Like the wind, either it can blow you off course or you can harness it to move yourself in the right direction. Chronic pain is just another obstacle that can be navigated past successfully with pain recovery. Rather than viewing this as a struggle, see it as a challenge and try to find enjoyment in the journey. All that is required is that you make progress toward balance each day; there is no point of completion. Striving for perfect balance, while an admirable goal, is not a realistic one. The seas may be calm for a while, but that rarely lasts. Human beings are fallible by nature, and trying to achieve perfection would actually cause imbalance.

As you become aware of circumstances in your life that are not in balance, resist the urge to correct by oversteering. There is no quick fix, and changes are most effective when made incrementally, with all four points being considered. Imbalance often results from being unduly harsh, so resist the urge to become discouraged, or to punish, blame, or feel shame.

These four points represent the whole of you and should not be viewed as disconnected or dealt with individually without regard for the complete picture. When all four points are working in conjunction with each other, they produce a synergistic effect that is greater than each point individually.

It is vital to be aware that situations you perceive as negative and challenging, such as death of a loved one, divorce, addiction, chronic pain, getting fired, or abuse can result in imbalance. Imbalance also can stem from situations you perceive as positive, such as job promotion, marriage, buying a house, or the birth of a child. Even a positive change in one point has the potential to disrupt your equilibrium. For example, if you put most of your effort into taking care of yourself physically, but don't pay attention to your thoughts, feelings, and spirit, you will be unbalanced. You might see your efforts as futile or believe they didn't work, but this is not what it means. It simply means you need to be aware that putting too much effort into one point and neglecting the others will result in overall imbalance.

The points are not a miracle cure for what ails you. Working toward balance requires diligence and persistent effort, and balancing the points can lead you to solutions for whatever you are experiencing and help you live a more meaningful and purposeful life.

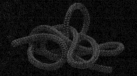

Part II

DISCOVER

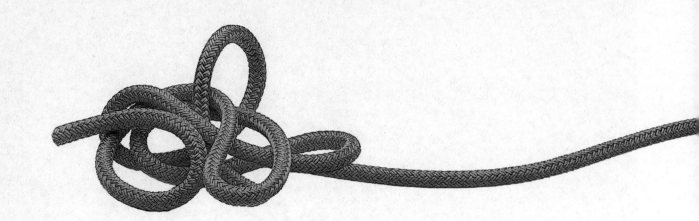

Physical Balance

We've described the key components of finding balance in pain recovery. Now we will examine each of the four points to help you discover where you are out of balance and give you the tools to work toward restoring balance. In this chapter we will look at the physical aspects of chronic pain and the body's recovery process. We will describe how pain signals interact with brain cells, resulting in the experience we call pain. We will also present information on medications commonly used to treat pain and on discontinuing medications. And finally, you will read about a number of nonmedication modalities that may help improve your physical condition and reduce your pain.

The Physical Experience of Pain

Pain as we experience it is the net effect of tissue disturbance, transmission to and from the brain, and extensive processing and modifying of the pain signal. With chronic pain, the signal and its transmission are often distorted. So pain levels increase, despite the fact that the injury has ended and the "need" for pain (protection, withdrawal, avoiding further injury) has passed.

Chronic pain is usually neuropathic, meaning associated with disturbances of the nervous system. Often the character of chronic pain differs from that of acute pain (called nociceptive pain), which is usually sharp, aching, or throbbing, and comes from sprains, fractures, burns, bruises, or other forms of tissue damage. Neuropathic pain is usually a burning sensation and may involve troublesome numbness. Neuropathic pain can have a lightning-bolt sensation or an electrical quality. With neuropathic pain, you may experience allodynia, which is pain from something that normally doesn't cause pain, such as light touch or a breeze across the skin. Also associated with neuropathic pain is hyperalgesia, meaning more pain than would normally be caused by a stimulus. This kind of pain may be difficult to localize, and the source of the pain may be widespread or changing.

Physical Extremes

Doing things that are good for you in an excessive manner is one extreme way to treat your body if you have chronic pain. For example, embarking on a vigorous course of exercise that might result in an injury, losing weight by starving yourself, or engaging in myriad activities that you haven't done before, such as acupuncture, massage, physical therapy, or chiropractic, spending money and time without developing a consistent plan.

Taking medications in excess of the recommended dosage and relying on them for your well-being, to the exclusion of exercise and stretching, is another common example of an extreme physical behavior.

Probably the most common extremes are patterns of unhealthy behaviors that cause damage to the body, including:

- Inactivity (which causes joints to stiffen and muscles to weaken and atrophy).

- Overeating or eating nonnutritious foods.

- Smoking and ingesting toxic substances.

- Not sleeping enough or sleeping too much (napping throughout the day, resulting in the inability to get extended, restful sleep at night).

- Taking mood-altering drugs.

The Pitfalls of Pain Management

Traditional pain management uses a multitude of interventions, including medications. This is a relatively new subspecialty of medicine. Most pain management specialists are trained as anesthesiologists, and usually go through a fellowship training program to learn to deal with chronic pain.

Opioid medications are the primary drugs used to treat chronic pain and are often the cornerstone of pain management. Unfortunately, they carry with them a potential for side effects, decrease in function, and in some cases the development of dependence and addiction. The side effects of opioids may include cloudy thinking, drowsiness, depression, and sleep disturbance. In women, opioids and chronic pain can lower estrogen levels, even leading to menopause and osteoporosis.

In some cases, increasing the dose of opioids can actually cause more pain, a phenomenon we described in Chapter Two known as opioid-induced hyperalgesia (OIH) that occurs in some people who are on long-term opioids. The proper treatment of OIH is to discontinue opioid medications so the brain can "reset" and eliminate the hyperalgesic effect of the drugs.

It may amaze you to know that there are no scientifically reliable studies that justify the use of opioids for longer than three months, even though that is standard operating procedure for treatment of chronic pain. There are a number of reasons for this disparity, but probably the best explanation is that opioids offer temporary relief to a permanent problem that is complex and difficult to treat. Doctors and drug companies have created an industry that promotes these powerful drugs for chronic pain, even though for many that is not the best course. Many patients have reported to us that they would never have started taking prescribed pain medication if they had known how much havoc it could wreak in their lives.

Additionally, painkillers are frequently prescribed in conjunction with other habit-forming medications, such as muscle relaxants (specifically Soma), stimulants used for sleepiness caused by the opioids, antianxiety drugs, and sleeping pills. The use of medications to treat the effects of other medications can be extremely frustrating for people with chronic pain and their families. You may end up on so many medications that your quality of life is severely compromised and you still have significant pain.

Not all medications are bad for you, but when taking any drugs, ask yourself what effect you are expecting and experiencing. Taking an extra vitamin for energy or a muscle relaxant to decrease anxiety is not addiction, but might underlie a thinking style that looks for a psychological effect from a drug. Many medications are not habit-forming and may be prescribed as part of a pain management plan; these include muscle relaxants, antiseizure medicines, and antidepressants. Each may be helpful, but if prescribed, should be taken under the supervision of a health professional knowledgeable about recovery and chronic pain. Furthermore, we recommend that you remain mindful of the effects of any medication that you are using, as well as its possible interactions with other prescription and over-the-counter medications.

Pain management also often includes invasive procedures such as injections (epidurals, facet blocks, and others) and surgeries, as well as nonmedication, nonsurgical techniques such as acupuncture, chiropractic, physical therapy, massage, and hydrotherapy.

You have most likely used a variety of substances and techniques to try to deal with your chronic pain. The following exercise concerns your treatment experiences up to this point.

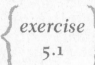

Pain Management Experience _____

List the medications that have been prescribed for you as well as those you have used that were not prescribed (put a P next to those prescribed and an N next to those not prescribed).

_____

_____

_____

_____

_____

Now list any substances you have used in addition to medications. Be as complete as you can and include alcohol, over-the-counter products, cigarettes, caffeine, and illegal drugs.

_____

_____

_____

_____

_____

Finally, list any treatment modalities or procedures you have used or undergone as part of your pain management. Indicate "+" or "−" as to whether they were helpful or not.

_____

_____

_____

_____

_____

JARED'S STORY

I entered this world in June of 1960 as happy as can be, or so I'm told. At age two, after some uncontrollable bleeding episodes, I was diagnosed with hemophilia B. From that point on, a "normal" life for me was a protected life, free from most activities that could cause me to bleed.

The treatment of hemophilia was in its early stages in the sixties. When I was young, the treatment was a lengthy hospital stay where I was given whole blood and fresh frozen plasma until the bleeding stopped. They also gave me codeine to ease the pain and calm me down, so at an early age, I was comfortably numb.

In my high school years I attended many weekend parties with alcohol, which I was able to "kick up a notch" with Tylenol No. 3; however, I remained functional and was able to graduate fourth in my class. I headed to college where my roommate loved drugs, and it didn't take much coaxing for me to join him. A few years later, following a car accident and a DWI, I wound up in an alcohol rehabilitation facility. When I got out, I attended twelve-step meetings but didn't get a sponsor and never did my fourth step. I eventually relapsed.

By 1985 I was a flight attendant for a major airline. This concerned my family because they felt there were too many temptations for someone with my history. As was usually the case, they were correct. In 1988, after a long night out, my colleagues dropped me off at my apartment, but I was locked out of my second-floor unit. I attempted to jump onto the deck from the ground and hit my head on an overhang. Eventually my roommate came home and let me in. She and her friends thought I was just drunk, until I was still lying there the next morning and couldn't be roused.

The next thing I remember was my mother and sisters crying over my bed as I came to after surgery. I had a brain bleed, a serious issue for anyone, but especially for someone with hemophilia. The neurosurgeon came in and told me I was fortunate that the injury occurred in the left frontal lobe, which controls emotions, and that I would have the "joie de vivre" (loosely translated, the "joy of life") for the rest of my life. Darvocet, Percocet, and Tylox became my new best friends following two brain surgeries to replace a bone flap that had become infected.

In the mid-nineties, I was being treated for chronic back pain that I'd been experiencing for several years. My doctor explained that there was a "wonderful new drug on the market to control pain—very safe and nonaddictive." My love affair with OxyContin began. By 2008, I was prescribed 400 mg twice a day. I was eating twelve 80 mg tablets at a time! I was powerless over my addiction, and my life was unmanageable.

I made a decision to stop the madness. I flew out West for treatment with the full, unwavering support of my family and the spiritual strength provided by my loving Higher Power. My back pain was between a five and a six on the one-to-ten pain scale. A Fentanyl patch was removed from my arm, and the process of healing began. During the course of my thirty-five-day stay in treatment, my hemophilia became "active." I had four separate acute bleeds, one which caused severe pain, but I got through it without the use of opioids. Practicing meditation, prayer, yoga, reiki, and other techniques helped me tremendously.

I now go to twelve-step meetings every day, I have a sponsor, and I'm looking forward to a "searching and fearless moral inventory." I'm good for today. Did I mention that since the third week of my treatment stay my back pain has been at a one? Hyperalgesia at its finest!

Prescription Pain Medications

We've described potential problems with taking opioids for chronic pain. Here are the names of medications in this class and other classes of drugs with habit-forming potential:

Table 5.1a

Mood-altering & Potentially Addictive Drugs (This list is not all-inclusive.)		
Type	**Brand Name**	**Generic Name**
Barbiturates	Fioricet/Codeine	Butalbital/Codeine/Acet/Caffeine
	Fiorinal	Butalbital/Aspirin/Caffeine
	Phenobarbital	Phenobarbital
Benzodiazepines	Ativan	Lorazepam
	Dalmane	Flurazepam
	Halcion	Triazolam
	Klonopin	Clonazepam
	Librium	Chlordiazepoxide
	Restoril	Temazepam
	Serax	Oxazepam
	Tranxene	Clorazepate Dipotassium
	Valium	Diazepam
	Xanax	Alprazolam
Hypnotics (for sleep)	Ambien	Zolpidem titrate
	Lunesta	Eszopiclone
	Sonata	Zaleplon
Muscle Relaxants	Soma	Carisoprodol
	Equagesic	Meprobamate/Aspirin
Opioids	Hycodan	Hydrocodone/Methylbromide
	Tussionex	Hydrocodone bit/Chlorpheneramine
	Actiq	Oral transmucosal fentanyl citrate
	Avinza	Morphine sulfate
	Demerol	Meperidine
	Dilaudid	Hydromorphone
	Duragesic	Fentanyl
	Kadian	Morphine sulfate
	Methadone	Methadone
	MS Contin	Morphine sulfate
	Oxycontin	Oxycodone
	Oxyfast	Oxycodone
	Percocet	Oxycodone/Acetaminophen
	Percodan	Oxycodone/Aspirin
	Tylox	Oxycodone/Acetaminophen
	Lorcet	Hydrocodone/Acetaminophen
	Lortab	Hydrocodone/Acetaminophen
	Norco	Hydrocodone/Acetaminophen
	Subutex	Buprenorphine hydrochloride
	Suboxone	Buprenorphine hydrochloride + naloxone

continued on page 67

Mood-altering & Potentially Addictive Drugs (continued)		
Type	**Brand Name**	**Generic Name**
Opioids	Tylenol/Codeine	Acetaminophen/Codeine
	Vicodin	Hydrocodone/Acetaminophen
	Vicoprofen	Hydrocodone/Ibuprofen
	Darvocet-N	Propoxyphene/Acetaminophen
	Darvon	Propoxyphene
	Stadol NS	Butorphanol tartrate
	Talwin NX	Pentazocine naloxone
Stimulants	Adderall	Amphetamine aspartate/Sulfate
	Dexedrine	Dextroamphetamine
	Concerta	Methylphenidate
	Ritalin	Methylphenidate

There are a number of nonopioid medications that are used to decrease pain. Here's a partial list:

Table 5.1b

Nonopioid Medications			
Drug Class		**Generic**	**Brand Name(s)**
Anticonvulsants		Gabapentin	Neurontin
		Topiramate	Topamax
		Carbemazepine	Tegretol
		Valproic Acid	Depakote
		Pregablin	Lyrica
Anti-depressants	*Tricyclics*	Amitryptilline	Elavil
		Desipramine	Norpramin
		Norpramine	Pamelor
	SSRI–SNRI	Venflaxine	Effexor
		Duloxetine	Cymbalta
NSAIDs	*COX 2s Traditional NSAIDs*	Celecoxib	Celebrex
		Ibuprofen	Advil, Motrin
		Naproxen	Naprosyn, Aleve
		Indomethacin	Indocin
		Nabunetone	Relafen
Muscle Relaxants		Methocarbamol	Robaxin
		Liorisal	Baclofen
		Metaxalone	Skelaxin
		Cyclobenzaprine	Flexeril
		Tizanadine	Xanaflex
Topicals		Capascins	Zostrix
		Lidocaine	Lidoderm patches

Discontinuing Medications

The safest way to discontinue medications is under medical supervision in an inpatient detox center. If you are unable to access such a setting, then you should consult with a medical provider to see how best to proceed. Depending on the dosage of the medications and how long you have taken them, your doctor may decide to have you stop the medication and substitute another or gradually wean you off of the medication(s) you are on. Either way, you are likely to experience increased pain as the dose decreases and/or stops.

The increased pain that occurs during withdrawal is temporary. If you are physically dependent on an opioid, you will not be able to discontinue your medications without temporarily experiencing increased pain and other withdrawal symptoms. Other symptoms you may experience include sweating, anxiety, agitation, skin crawling, runny nose, yawning, nausea, vomiting, diarrhea, and insomnia.

It is important to remember that these symptoms will pass and may be decreased by prescription medications including clonidine, phenobarbital, hydroxyzine, and sleep aids. Sometimes major tranquilizers (antipsychotic drugs) such as Seroquel (quetiapine) or Risperdal (risperidone) will be indicated for severe agitation. Please discuss all of these with your physician.

Therapies for Pain Relief

Be mindful of what works best (when, how, etc.) for your pain while you are trying many approaches. For example, for some, applying heat followed by cold to the painful area works best. Other people do better with just heat or cold alone. For still others, usually those with neuropathic or nerve pain, their pain is aggravated by the application of either heat or cold. Some things work as soon as you do them, like acupuncture and massage. Others may initially make your discomfort worse, like physical therapy or movement modalities, but if you continue to do them they will result in real, lasting improvement.

{ *exercise* 5.2 }

*Evaluating Your Pain*_____

1. Write about the body part(s) that are affected by your chronic pain.

_____

_____

_____

_____

2. What makes the painful sensation worse?

_____

_____

_____

3. What makes it better?

_____

_____

_____

_____

Choosing Practitioners and Techniques

It is important when pursuing therapies to choose qualified and knowledgeable practitioners to ensure you are receiving the best care. We also recommend informing your doctor of any therapies you are considering. Be careful not to exceed your capabilities and injure yourself, though you may be able to gently "push yourself" through difficult exercise. Just keep in mind a common saying in some twelve-step programs: "Easy does it." We have listed some basic information on several modalities that have been shown to be beneficial for chronic pain. As you will see, many of these modalities are about balancing your mind, body, emotions, and spirit.

EXERCISE

When you are in pain, you may feel inclined to rest and avoid exercise; however, exercise is one of the best things you can do to ultimately reduce your pain. The danger of inactivity is that your body becomes deconditioned, which can add substantially to your perception and experience of pain. Studies have shown that regular and sustained physical activity is beneficial to virtually every system in the body. During exercise your body releases chemicals called endorphins, which naturally relieve pain and also help to lessen anxiety and depression. The four major types of exercise are cardiovascular, strength training, balance, and stretching.

Some other benefits of regular exercise include:

> ❧ **Helping you maintain a healthy weight.** Dropping extra pounds can lessen the stress you place on your joints, which is one way to ease bone pain.

ns flexibility, you are less likely to strain

stantially to chronic pain.

nger you are, the better your muscles

. The healthier the muscle, the less pain

improves your mood and fights pain by

e brain. It is a natural sleep regulator, and

tion of pain.

eart and circulatory system. Exercise

art attack, and diabetes. It also reduces high

results in improved moods and increased

your dopamine level and add strength to all

ses to fight chronic pain, which may have

e.

> Before beginning any exercise program, you should consult with your doctor to be sure the exercises are appropriate and helpful for your specific situation.

FOODS AND NUTRITION

What we eat every day has a profound effect on how we feel. Our foods play a major role in our health and well-being. According to Dr. Neal Barnard, author of *Foods That Fight Pain*, foods fight pain in four distinct ways:

- They can reduce damage at the site of an injury.

- They work inside the brain to reduce pain sensitivity.

- They act as painkillers on nerves.

- They help our bodies fight inflammation.

A healthy diet can extend our lives and help us fight many chronic diseases that often lead to chronic pain or make it worse. Without a doubt, being and feeling healthy helps us fight pain sensations.

RECOMMENDED READING

Foods That Fight Pain, by Neal Barnard, MD; Three Rivers Press.

PHYSICAL THERAPY

Physical therapy (PT) is the treatment, prevention, and management of movement disorders arising from conditions and diseases. A good PT program with a qualified therapist can help you reduce discomfort, increase flexibility, and improve function. PT may encompass techniques such as manipulation, traction, massage, therapeutic exercise, functional training, education, and counseling about movement and healthy body mechanics. Physical therapists use ice, heat, electrical currents, and a variety of newer techniques to relieve adhesions (e.g., Graston technique, active release techniques) and to decrease sympathetic tone (e.g., Primal Reflex Release Technique).

Because each individual is different, physical therapists design programs specifically for each person. These programs usually also include goal-setting and monitoring of progress. Achieving goals helps boost your confidence and reinforce your sense of self-efficacy, factors that are closely linked to positive outcomes in chronic pain treatment.

PILATES

Pilates is an innovative system of mind-body exercise developed by Joseph Pilates in the early 1900s. It was designed to build strength and improve flexibility without adding bulk. The Pilates method, as well as the specially-designed apparatus used with the exercises, focuses on core postural muscles that keep the body balanced and are essential to support the spine. Pilates teaches awareness of neutral spine alignment and strengthens the muscles that support this alignment. The alignment helps treat and prevent back pain and reduces the potential for injury. Controlled breathing and concentration are also an essential element of Pilates, making it a mind-body workout and an effective way to reduce stress and promote relaxation.

TENS

TENS means transcutaneous electrical nerve stimulation. TENS units are small, battery-powered devices that produce a vibration or signal intended to interrupt pain transmissions from nerves before they reach the brain. TENS units (or electrical stimulators) can be implanted and operated with small controls that send signals through the skin into the muscles. TENS is considered to be the electrical equivalent of portable acupuncture or acupressure.

TENS falls into a treatment category called "hyperstimulation analgesia." These treatments include vibration, acupressure, acupuncture, and massage. There are two theories practitioners use to explain how TENS works. The first is the gate theory that says nerves can carry only one signal at a time, and the TENS signal overrides the pain signal, in effect closing the gate on pain transmissions before they can reach the brain. The second theory is the endorphin theory that claims TENS stimulates the body's production of natural painkillers, giving users relief.

COMPLEMENTARY AND ALTERNATIVE MEDICINE (CAM)

Chronic pain often leads people to areas outside of conventional Western medicine. More and more Americans are trying complementary and alternative treatments for their ailments, and this is especially true for those in chronic pain. According to a study in the *Journal of the American Medical Association,* 40 percent of Americans and more than two-thirds of the world population use complementary or alternative therapies. The quality of research supporting CAM varies from therapy to therapy. As with any treatment approach, use of CAM should be discussed with your doctor.

Acupuncture

Practitioners of acupuncture believe illness, including chronic pain, is due to imbalances of energy in the body. Acupuncture is a component of traditional Chinese medicine in which the body is seen as a balance of two opposing and inseparable forces or energy—yin and yang. Yin represents cold, slow, or passive aspects of the person, while yang represents hot, excited, or active aspects. This energy is also known as chi. Health is achieved through balancing of yin and yang, and disease is caused by an imbalance of these forces, leading to a blockage in the flow of chi.

In acupuncture, hair-thin steel needles are inserted into the body to stimulate fourteen energy-carrying channels to correct the imbalances. Acupuncture is thought to relieve pain by increasing the release of endorphins. Acupuncture is effective at treating chronic pain including back, neck, and muscle pain, headache, facial pain, arthritis, and shingles.

Aromatherapy

Aromatherapy literally means the therapeutic use of scents to change moods. Essential oils distilled from plants, flowers, trees, bark, grasses, seeds, and fruits are used to treat a variety of ailments including fatigue, tension, stress, and, most importantly here, pain.

Aromatherapy is also one of the fastest-growing natural remedies being used today. It works by awakening and strengthening the self-healing ability of the body. Smells can have a profound effect on our sense of well-being and body balance. The essential oils used in aromatherapy are antiseptic, antidepressant, antiviral, anti-inflammatory, detoxifying, expectorant, and analgesic.

Ayurveda

Ayurveda medical practitioners believe we're all born in a state of balance. This balance is thrown out of whack by the processes of life. These disruptions can be physical, emotional, spiritual, or combinations of all these. This is much like pain recovery. In Ayurveda, an individual's prakriti, or essential "constitution," is considered to be a unique combination of physical and psychological characteristics, as well as ways in which the body's constitution functions.

Three qualities called doshas form important characteristics of the body and control the body's activities. The doshas are called by their original Sanskrit names: vata, pitta, and kapha. Each dosha is associated with a certain body type and personality type. An imbalance in any dosha may be caused by an unhealthy lifestyle or diet, too much or too little mental and physical exertion, improper digestion, or problems with how the body eliminates waste products. A person's health will be good if he or she returns to balance and has a wholesome interaction with the environment.

Biofeedback

Biofeedback is a technique that can help you learn to control some normally involuntary processes by raising your awareness of signals from your body. This is accomplished using specialized equipment that allows you to monitor bodily functions such as blood pressure, heart rate, muscle tension, sweat gland activity, and skin temperature. Biofeedback may be beneficial in treating your chronic pain because it harnesses the power of the mind to improve your condition and puts you in control of your own pain perception and healing. In general, those who benefit most from biofeedback have conditions that are brought on or made worse by stress.

Body Scan/Meditation

One specific meditative practice is called the body scan, which is adapted from an ancient Burmese practice. Jon Kabat-Zinn, Ph.D., writes in *Full Catastrophe Living* that the body scan "is an effective technique for developing both concentration and flexibility of attention simultaneously. It involves lying on your back and moving your mind through the different regions of your body." This guided meditation encourages you to scan through your body much like a CT scan machine might. One key is to simply notice the sensation without judging it. It utilizes the breath to affect and decrease tension and pain. Each time you encounter these feelings you can replace them with a sense of spaciousness, relaxation, and freedom.

Chi Kung (Qigong)

Chi Kung, also known as Qigong, is a Chinese practice that integrates physical postures, breathing exercises, and mental focus. The word "Chi" means life force or vital energy, and "Kung" means skill achieved through consistent practice. Practitioners of Chi Kung believe most physical problems, including pain and diseases, are related to imbalances of vital energy fields, and that by restoring your internal/external balance you can maintain health and promote healing and vitality. Research has confirmed many of the benefits of the practice.

Chi Kung is moving meditation, and is a very gentle form of exercise that can be practiced by all age groups and can be easily modified for those with physical challenges. Specific exercises help release negative energy and focus on specific areas of the body, such as the spine. With consistent practice, Chi Kung can help you develop a more positive outlook, restore balance, and enhance quality of life.

Chiropractic

Chiropractic therapy diagnoses and treats problems involving nerves, bones, muscles, and joints. Chiropractors believe that manipulation of muscles, the spine, and other joints helps the body heal itself. Chiropractic medicine is the third largest health profession in the Western world. More than twenty million people are treated each year.

Manipulation is the primary treatment offered by chiropractors, although there are other therapies offered including massage and prescribed exercises. Chiropractors sometimes use various tests to help with their diagnoses such as X-rays, blood tests, and blood pressure readings.

Although chiropractic medicine has a lot in common with other health professions, it is unique in its belief that spinal misalignment is the cause of most forms of illness. Many people visit a chiropractor for a specific problem; however, chiropractors report that their manipulations benefit the person's health in a general way. There are hundreds of different techniques and methods of manipulation used by chiropractors to treat as many conditions. Research has shown that chiropractic medicine is effective in many cases to reduce and treat acute and chronic back pain. It also has been shown to help many painful conditions including frozen shoulder, muscle spasms, and carpal tunnel syndrome.

Herbs

More and more people have found that using herbal painkillers has fewer side effects and long-term risks than traditional medicines. Research has shown that some herbal medicines not only help relieve pain, but also can attack some of the underlying causes of the pain. One of the most common herbal medicines is white willow bark. It has been used for centuries to relieve pain. It can help reduce acute or chronic pain in the back, joints, teeth, and head.

Other herbs used to fight pain include feverfew, ginger, cat's claw, cayenne, eucalyptus, aloe vera, lobelia, neem, yellow dock, passion flower, hops, and wood betony.

Herbs technically are drugs and should be treated as such. Some can produce side effects and carry risks when not taken responsibly. It is always important to consult with your doctor and pharmacist before taking any herbal preparations since they can have reactions with your other medications. Also, many herbal preparations are made with an alcohol base. These should not be taken by someone in recovery. Always make sure you read labels for warnings and ingredients and seek professional advice before taking herbal products.

Hypnotherapy

Hypnotherapy uses concentration, relaxation, and focused attention to attain a heightened state of awareness called a trance or hypnotic state. The person in the trance becomes able to block out outside stimuli and concentrate on specific tasks or thoughts. It is used to help people perceive stimuli differently, such as by blocking the perception of pain.

Hypnotherapy addresses both physical and mental causes of pain. Therapists say that hypnotherapy helps people regulate the type, strength, and amount of pain signals that reach the brain. People can reprogram their bodies to lessen the amount of pain-inducing chemicals released. Conversely, people also can learn to regulate the amount of pain-relieving endorphins. The goal of hypnotherapy in relation to chronic pain is to produce deep relaxation to lower the fear, tension, and anxiety that usually accompany pain.

Hydrotherapy/Hydromassage

Hydrotherapy involves the therapeutic use of water to maintain health and to treat and prevent disease. According to proponents, there is no medicine on the market that can rival the beneficial physiological effects of water. Maintaining hydration is necessary for the function of all vital organs. Benefits of hydrotherapy include helping with sleep, controlling temperature, providing derivative pain relief, and acting as an anticonvulsant. Hydromassage is a popular treatment that uses water to apply massage techniques. This therapy can relieve muscle pain and tension, improve circulation, promote relaxation, and reduce stress and anxiety.

Magnet Therapy

Magnets have been used for centuries to treat a variety of conditions including arthritis, painful swollen joints, and blood diseases. Most modern medical practitioners are uncommitted on magnetic therapy. Even for practitioners who insist magnets relieve pain, why they work is still a mystery. Some theorize that magnets may change how cells function, change how the brain processes pain, raise the temperature of the area being treated by the magnets, restore the equilibrium between cell growth and death, change how nerves transmit pain signals, and/or have an effect on the iron content in blood. In general, practitioners place magnets with a constant flow of energy in contact with the area of the body they wish to affect. This "static magnet treatment" is used in a number of different ways, including having the magnets in clothing, belts, jewelry, and beds.

Massage

As a treatment, massage is used in conventional medicine as well as in CAM. The basic goal of the massage therapist is to increase the flow of blood and oxygen to a specific area of the body, relax and warm the soft tissues, and decrease pain by pressing, rubbing, and moving soft muscles and other tissues, primarily using the hands and fingers.

People use massage for any number of reasons and health-related purposes including for general wellness, for rehabilitation, to increase relaxation, to decrease stress, to help alleviate feelings of depression or anxiety, and to relieve pain. There is no doubt that a soothing massage can ease the pain of a long day and soothe achy joints and muscles.

A variety of reasons are cited for why massage is an effective treatment for chronic pain. Some believe that rubbing and stroking may override and block painful signals from reaching the brain. A number of practitioners believe that massage lessens many of the factors that contribute to the sense of pain, including stress, muscle tension, and spasm, and pain itself is then eased. They say that since pain and tension decrease blood circulation and massage increases it, manipulation has a negating effect on painful areas. Massage helps stimulate "feel-good" areas of the brain, which produces more of its natural opioid painkillers.

Many massage techniques can be temporarily painful, as the weight of the therapist's body puts pressure on muscles, joints, and tendons to "release" them, resulting in reduction of pain. This is another example of long-term gains from short-term increase in discomfort.

Music Therapy

Music therapy is the clinical use of music to treat patients with physical, psychological, cognitive, and social functioning issues. It is a powerful and noninvasive method to reduce pain, anxiety, and depression. The treatment is for patients of all ages, with outcomes based on the individual's emotional, cognitive, and interpersonal responsiveness to the music and/or therapy relationship.

As a form of sensory stimulation, music provokes responses based on familiarity, predictability, and feelings of security. Therapists use musical activities, both instrumental and vocal, to cause changes in a patient's condition. Music treatment has been used to reduce stress and anxiety, help patients manage pain without drugs, and encourage positive changes in mood and emotional states. Music helps patients deal with pain by improving respiration, lowering blood pressure, improving heart output, and easing muscle tension.

Reflexology

Reflexology promotes healing through stimulation of points in the hands and feet, which are divided into zones that correspond to parts of the body. This natural therapy is said to help identify blockages, reduce stress and tension, promote healing and relaxation, improve circulation, eliminate toxins, and restore equilibrium. The treatment is not painful, and most people find it relaxing. Reflexology can be beneficial for many conditions and for improving general health and well-being.

Reiki

Reiki promotes good health through relaxation, stress relief, and pain management. In reiki, "universal life-force energy" is transmitted through the hands of a therapist from the vast pool of energy that abounds in the universe. Also called "palm healing" and "energy medicine," reiki is made up of two Japanese words; "rei," meaning universal spirit or spiritual wisdom, and "ki," meaning energy or life-force energy.

In CAM, energy therapies are based on the assumption that illness and pain are caused by disturbances in a person's energy. Reiki practitioners seek to improve the flow and balance of positive energy and reduce negative energy in a way that is beneficial to clients. The energy flows wherever it is needed and often is reported as a tingling in the body. Most report being extremely relaxed after a reiki treatment.

Reiki treatments have been used to reduce chronic pain, help with recovery from anesthesia and surgery, improve immunity, improve mental clarity, and lower a person's heart rate. Reiki practitioners often report clients experiencing a "cleansing crisis" after a session, in which they have feelings of nausea, tiredness, or weakness because of the release of energy toxins.

Yoga

Yoga is a Sanskrit word meaning "union." It can be thought of as a form of exercise developed over thousands of years in India. It promotes health and happiness by working on the mind, body, and spirit. Yoga is being used more and more as a treatment modality. Where the techniques and benefits of yoga were once in doubt as a therapy, physicians are now turning to it as a viable treatment for many different conditions, including pain. Study after study has shown that for many people, yoga is one of the most effective treatments for increasing mobility and reducing pain.

Yoga works on stretching and strengthening the body. By increasing strength, improving flexibility, and ridding the body of muscle tension, a person can bring their body into balance and ease their pain. Practicing yoga can allow someone to focus on positive aspects of life, as opposed to focusing strictly on pain. Deep breathing has physical and psychological benefits that can help calm the extreme emotional effects of chronic pain. There are now hundreds, if not thousands, of different "styles" of yoga, each promoting a different path to similar conclusions.

{ *exercise* 5·3 } *Maintaining Physical Balance* _____

Write a list of balancing physical behaviors for your maintenance program. Be specific and include resources and practitioners that have been helpful in the past.

_____
_____
_____
_____
_____
_____

{ *exercise* 5·4 } *Crisis Intervention* _____

Write a list of crisis intervention behaviors you might use if you have a flare-up of pain.

_____
_____
_____
_____
_____
_____

ALTERED BODY IMAGE

Since we are discussing the body, it is significant to address the fact that many with chronic pain have an altered body image (ABI). We want to remind you that you are still the same person inside that you were before you had chronic pain. Try learning new ways to do at least some of the things you enjoyed before. You may need to be creative. Don't limit yourself with the label of "disabled." The focus should no longer be on chronic pain and what you can't do, but rather on enhancing function and doing what you can.

Sexuality

Chronic pain can interfere with a healthy sex life in a number of ways. You may have difficulty being sexual because your self-esteem has plummeted and you feel bad about yourself. Changing roles or household patterns because of chronic pain may also affect sexuality. Another common problem is anticipation or fear of pain, which can interfere with performance or act as a trigger in causing you to avoid sex.

Intercourse may be physically uncomfortable for a person in pain. Opioids and other painkillers can cause physiological changes that affect sexual functioning. According to studies, in men, opioids can lower testosterone levels, suppress sexual function, and cause erectile dysfunction. They can also contribute to low libido and difficulty with orgasm in both sexes. If you have chronic pain and take medications for depression such as Prozac (fluoxetine), Zoloft (sertraline), or others, side effects in both men and women may include decreased sex drive and difficulty reaching orgasm.

There is no need to be celibate or ashamed. If these issues affect you, we encourage you to talk to your doctor, counselor, and sexual partner. If your doctor does not bring it up, ask about the side effects of your medication as a way to start the conversation. A pain journal may be useful when you are at home for jotting down points and reflecting on when you were intimate with your partner. At what point did your pain occur, and what was going on when your pain subsided? Once your doctor has a clear picture, he or she can work on helping you to plan for alleviating pain during sexual activity.

Sexual activity is a normal part of intimacy and need not be given up. Reigniting intimacy can actually help reduce pain and suffering. During orgasm, the body floods with endorphins, and this helps relieve pain. Trying different positions or activities other than traditional intercourse may be satisfying and enhance intimacy without causing pain, so we encourage you to think creatively. Express your limitations and desires to your partner. Tell your partner what is pleasurable and what is not. Communication is the key, and may best be accomplished outside the bedroom.

> Remember, your loved ones are not mind readers.
> Healthy communication is the key to intimacy.

The body is one of the cornerstones of the experience of pain; therefore, balancing our physical life is a fundamental component of pain recovery. There are many ways to impact physical balance and enhance pain recovery. Next we will look at the other three points of balance—mental, emotional, and spiritual.

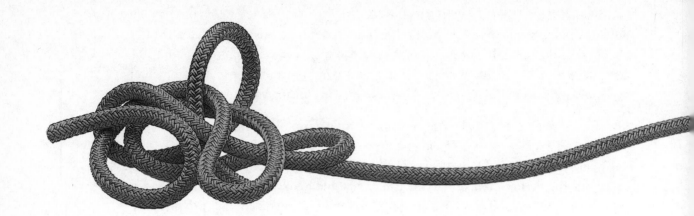

6

Mental Balance

When you look at the word "thought" or "think," what comes to mind? There's the first clue—we conceptualize a thought in our mind. In this chapter we will explore the point of balance most directly related to our minds and the net product of our minds' work—our thoughts. Your thoughts have a powerful influence on the pain you experience, as well as on how you respond to it. And how you respond to pain can either promote recovery or hinder it.

According to Merriam-Webster's Collegiate Dictionary, thought is "...reasoning power; the power to imagine; a developed intention or plan; or something (as an opinion or belief) in the mind..."* Thoughts and thinking are based on considering information that we come in contact with, analyzing this information, and forming conclusions as to what it means. Where do our thoughts come from? How are they formed and changed? Before we discuss the mechanics of thought, we will present extremes of thought common to people with chronic pain, as well as those with addiction. Extreme thinking creates or significantly contributes to the experience of pain and to an overall lack of balance in our lives.

Unchallenged, unhealthy thoughts create a burden
too heavy for you to carry.

Extremes of Thinking

One extreme style of thinking is to virtually "skip over" thoughts entirely (think too little). As a result, emotions are expressed in uncontrolled and sometimes frightening ways. If this is so for you, you may react to situations immediately, emotionally, and

*By permission. From Merriam-Webster's Collegiate® Dictionary, 11th Edition, ©2008 by Merriam-Webster, Incorporated (www.Merriam-Webster.com).

impulsively, rather than by thinking logically and acting based on consideration of the needs of the situation and selecting from available options.

Another extreme is to intellectualize situations (think too much). Ideas are king, and thinking is respected and even revered, while emotions are considered messy or unsafe, and their expression is suppressed, discouraged, minimized, or swept aside. You approach all situations intellectually and seek logical solutions, often to the neglect of appropriate emotional considerations. In extreme intellectualized thinking, excessive emphasis on thoughts and obsessive thinking about every possible option effectively paralyze decision making and prevent necessary action from taking place.

In the case of either of these extremes, you are "underthinking"—unaware of your thoughts—or "overthinking"—consumed by your thoughts.

Still another extreme of thought is to believe that everything will be fine no matter what. This can be mislabeled as positive thinking, but it's really a potentially dangerous way of thinking that flies in the face of reality—commonly referred to as denial. In this case, the pendulum swings to the extreme of not seeing reality as it truly is. This can lead to consequences such as underestimating potential problems, ignoring negative realities, not taking care of yourself, and placing yourself in risky situations. For example, you truly don't see the nature of the drug problem that has developed.

On the other side of this spectrum is thinking that everything is lousy and always will be, regardless of what happens. Chronic negative thinking actually makes "bad" situations worse. You may ruminate (go over and over a situation in your mind, replaying it unproductively) or magnify the negative, exaggerating the significance of something that occurred and turning what was really only a small problem into a major disaster in your mind. By focusing on the negative aspects of your experience—for example, the initial injury that started your pain—you actually make your life more negative. Your thoughts have the capacity to make you miserable. Negative thinking can be especially insidious, feeding on itself, with the potential to become a self-fulfilling prophecy. Because the effects of chronic pain are generally so unpleasant, it is relatively easy for you to become trapped in a web of negativity from which it can be difficult to escape.

Your thinking may or may not take you to these extremes, but having chronic pain or addiction or both typically includes experiencing various degrees of distorted, out-of-balance thinking. Imbalance in thinking can cause imbalances in emotional, physical, and spiritual functioning.

Thinking about Thinking

Have you ever considered why you think what you think? Does it seem like your thoughts are who you are? The reality is that nothing could be further from the truth. Your thoughts are part of you, but only a part of the much greater whole. Descartes, a famous philosopher, said, "I think, therefore I am." This statement represented a step forward in the evolution of Western philosophy. However, in suggesting there is no separation between people and their thoughts, it also has done a disservice to our understanding of the relationship between our thoughts and who we *are*. Because they occur so automatically and seem so natural, we may become so closely identified with our thoughts that we believe there is no separation: Our thoughts are us and we are our thoughts. And yet, the reality is that thoughts are mental products generated in our brain.

We also tend to believe in the inherent truth or accuracy of our thoughts, believing "I think it, therefore it is true." Assuming our thoughts are facts—that they are all true and valid without examination—is one of the reasons we find ourselves out of balance.

Before emotion or action takes place in any situation, a thought process occurs; but it can happen so quickly and automatically that you're not consciously aware of it. These seemingly natural, automatic thoughts are also known as "self-talk"—the things you tell yourself about what is occurring that also define your beliefs about those events. While you may be powerless over the self-talk that first enters your mind, you are not powerless over what you do in response to it. You can detach from your thoughts—observe them, question their accuracy, dispute or talk back to them, and, ultimately, change them.

Self-Talk _____

{ *exercise* 6.1 }

Identify your automatic thoughts or self-talk about your chronic pain.

{example: Because I am not able to manage my pain, it must mean that I am weak.}

_____
_____
_____
_____
_____
_____

Now examine each thought and describe whether it is true or not.

_____

_____

_____

_____

_____

_____

What things have you done as a result of your thoughts that have made your pain worse?

_____

_____

_____

_____

_____

In pain recovery, we learn that we are not what we think. We can observe our thoughts and we can dispute them by not buying everything they are trying to sell us. Paying attention to your thought process and consciously questioning and challenging your thinking is an indication of mental balance. The more consciously aware of this process you can become, the more you will be able to develop the capacity to intentionally adjust your thinking and self-talk to cope with your pain more effectively and improve your functioning.

Progress toward healing and recovery from chronic pain also requires accepting that you cannot *control* your thoughts, but you can *modify* and *redirect* them. This requires the willingness to surrender, and the action of challenging and redirecting your thoughts in order to achieve balance.

Not everything you think is necessarily true or accurate.

Learning to view and respond to your thoughts differently will require going through a process of adjustment. The process is a lot like that of getting a new pair of shoes after having had the old ones for a very long time. The old shoes fit us like a glove; the leather has molded itself to fit the shape of our feet precisely. They have been so comfortable for so long that we don't want to part with them. And yet, they no longer work for us. They are dirty and torn, and the sole has no grip left. It is clear to most everyone but us that our shoes are a mess and we need new ones.

But we don't want new shoes; we like the ones we have just fine. We think if everyone would just leave us alone and let us wear our tattered shoes, everything would be fine. But, deep down, we know otherwise. A part of us desperately wants to hold onto the old shoes because we are so used to them that we can't imagine life without them, while another part of us knows that the old shoes aren't working any longer and we really do need new ones. We fear what life will be like without our old shoes. We think that there is no way new shoes could possibly fit us as well or be as comfortable as our old ones. Finally, our feet become so battered, bruised, and blistered that we can no longer deny to ourselves that we need new shoes. Perhaps with the help and support of family and/or significant others, we get a new pair of shoes. At first they are unfamiliar and feel awkward; they're stiff and somewhat uncomfortable.

However, if we can tolerate the initial discomfort and we practice wearing them, gradually, over time, they begin to feel more comfortable. The process of breaking in these new shoes does not happen as fast or as easily as we want it to. Yet, by our continuing to wear them one day at a time, it does happen. Eventually, the new shoes become even more comfortable than the old ones. Moreover, they provide the support our feet need and keep them warm and dry.

Holding and Changing _____

{ *exercise* 6.2 }

Write about a pattern of thinking you have developed that is not helpful to you but that you do not want to change (your old shoes—seemingly comfortable).

_____

_____

_____

_____

_____

Why do you insist on holding onto those thoughts?

_____

_____

_____

_____

_____

How can you change these thoughts to be more helpful (what will it take to get a new pair of shoes)?

_____

_____

_____

_____

How Self-Defeating Thoughts Create Imbalance

Imbalances of thought, wherein our minds approach what is happening in our external reality in an inaccurate way, are a common phenomenon. Our minds have the responsibility and challenge of making sense of our experience in the world so that we can understand it. Depending on external circumstances and internal influences, the mind can easily make errors in interpreting our experiences, thus throwing us out of balance.

The mechanics of thinking can be significantly distorted by pain and pain medications. Pain can take up so much space in our thinking that little room is left for the healthy consideration of available options. Opioid pain medications can dull and cloud the thought process, making imbalanced thinking, twisted beliefs, and inaccurate interpretations of events and situations much more likely.

The following sections focus on some specific and common imbalances in thinking that may be contributing to your suffering. These self-defeating thoughts have the potential to sabotage your efforts to achieve pain recovery.

SELF-ESTEEM/SELF-IMAGE

The progressive nature of chronic pain and addiction leads you to be less able to do things you once did with ease. Ongoing use of opioids and other medications leads to impaired thought processes. As this happens, your self-image and self-talk can become increasingly negative and focus nearly exclusively on your losses and deficits. This may happen gradually enough that you are unaware of the changes in your thinking and the way you view yourself. It is not unusual to be defensive about this and be unwilling or unable to admit to yourself and others how badly you are feeling about yourself. You may overcompensate by trying to be perfect at the things you can do and pointing this out to others. Or you may withdraw, and even stop trying altogether, since having a "normal life" may seem impossible. The pain-recovery process encourages you to look specifically at what you think and feel about yourself—your abilities, your limits, and what matters to you. This is part of the process of change that will lead you back to balance and the life you want to live.

You may have become so identified with your chronic pain that it becomes part of your core identity; you begin to think of yourself as a "victim," and pain becomes who you are rather than an experience that you sometimes have. The attention, concern, and sympathy you often receive from medical professionals, family members, and significant others serves to reinforce this self-perception and identification as a sufferer and/or victim, thus expanding the vicious-circle dynamic from how you relate to your own thoughts and emotions to the way you relate to others and to the world.

Many people who live with chronic pain can, over time, come to define their sense of self in terms of their pain and impaired functioning. "I used to be able to do this or that" or "I used to provide better for my family" have roots in reality for some, but can also equate to "I am very weak" or "I'm no longer valuable to my loved ones." Maintaining a balanced sense of self is essential to overall health. From a self-image standpoint, this might take the form of "I have lots of pain to deal with, and I'm developing tools to recover. I'm grateful for what I can do. In spite of my challenges, I have the ability to have a meaningful life, and it all begins with the way I think about myself."

Your Self-Image _____ { *exercise* 6.3 }

List some words you use to describe yourself.

_____
_____
_____
_____
_____

What changes can you make in your thoughts to improve your self-image?

_____
_____
_____
_____
_____

DISCOUNTING THE POSITIVE

As we've discussed, the sheer discomfort of chronic pain often results in negative thought patterns. One form these thoughts can take is to ignore, dismiss, or otherwise not be aware of anything remotely positive about this situation, whatever it may be. With or without your knowledge, you end up focusing all your conscious attention and energy on the negative aspects of the situation. For example, you hear from ten people how well you seem to be doing, while a single person tells you, for whatever reason, that you don't seem to be doing well. Rather than believe the ten people with positive views, you are certain that the one negative perspective is correct. In addition to feeding your negativity, this can also serve the self-defeating purpose of confirming what you believe about yourself—that you are not doing well. We find evidence in real events to support the position we've already taken.

In order to counteract this and reestablish balanced thinking, it is essential to keep in mind that nearly all situations and events have both positive and negative characteristics. Sometimes you may have to look a little harder or even do some work to locate the positive, but if you search for it, you will find it. Something else you can do to counteract this form of thinking is to identify things or people you are grateful for. Practicing expressing gratitude can improve mood and measurably increase the experience of happiness.

{ *exercise* 6.4 }

Transforming Negatives to Positives _____

Describe the negative aspects of your pain.

_____

_____

_____

_____

Now take a closer look and identify some positive characteristics about it.

_____

_____

_____

_____

Identify things or people you are grateful for and briefly describe the reason(s) for your gratitude.

_____

_____

_____

_____

MAKING MOUNTAINS OUT OF MOLEHILLS

Some of us have a tendency to get caught up in spinning elaborate scenarios related to events that may never actually occur, and spend considerable time and emotional energy looking for potential trouble, as well as for solutions to problems that don't exist. For instance, you sense pain in a specific area of your body that may be uncomfortable, but in and of itself is not that big a deal. However, your self-talk tells you, "This is horrible! It's going to spread to my entire body. I'll be in intense pain and have to spend the day, maybe even several days, in bed."

Thinking that catastrophe is upon you or inevitable has considerable influence on your experience of pain and your perceived options. The first step in interrupting this process is to become aware of it and realize what you are thinking. Only then can you make an informed decision about how you want and need to proceed based on the options available.

Keeping Things in Perspective _____ { *exercise* 6.5 }

Describe a situation where your thinking about your pain caused you to make things worse for yourself.

_____

_____

_____

_____

Describe how you can think differently in order to regain balance (be as specific as you can).

_____

_____

_____

_____

"BLACK-AND-WHITE" THINKING

Thinking in "either/or" terms, where things are the complete opposite of one another with nothing in between, creates imbalance in thinking by viewing events, situations, and people (including yourself) in one of only two mutually exclusive ways: all good or all bad. Everything is either "great" or it's "horrible." Self-perception tends to be based on the extremes of "I am perfect"/"I am a total failure" or "I am in constant pain"/"I must be totally pain-free."

Your thinking can also shift from one extreme to the other, depending on circumstances. In this thought pattern there is no middle ground. In fact, most of reality occurs somewhere in the middle, between the black and white and within those many shades of gray. When you are unable to see and appreciate this middle ground, you end up missing much of the richness and subtlety of life.

You can regain balance by becoming consciously aware of this tendency, checking your thought process and noticing when you are thinking in black-and-white terms. This awareness will provide the opportunity to look for the middle ground, the shades of gray that you are missing. Realistically, you are probably not in pain all of the time, and you are probably not completely comfortable all or none of the time.

{ *exercise* 6.6 } *Seeing the Shades of Gray* _____

Describe when you have engaged in black-and-white thinking.

_____
_____
_____
_____

Now, identify the shades of gray that exist between the two extremes.

_____
_____
_____
_____

EXPECTATIONS OF YOURSELF AND OTHERS

Everyone has beliefs about how things *should* be in relation to themselves, to others, and to the world. Expectations usually involve judging yourself, others, and situations against specific standards for behavior and reality that you've created in your mind. Sometimes these expectations become imperatives, such as "Things *must* be the way I want them to be." Whenever you think in terms of how people or situations should be, you set yourself up for disappointment.

When you don't perform as you think you should; when others don't act as you think they should; when situations don't turn out as you think they should, the resulting emotions are likely to include guilt, shame, frustration, hurt, and anger. For people struggling with chronic pain, this can create serious imbalances in thinking along the lines of: "It's not fair that I got hurt and now I can't work. I should be able to do all the things I used to do. This shouldn't have happened and I should not have to be in pain. But since I'm in pain, everyone should just let me take my pain medication however I want to in order to feel better!"

A solution to restore balanced thinking when you're caught up in expectations is to consciously separate what you may want from the reality of the situation. It's normal, natural, and understandable to want things the way you want them. But mental balance and pain recovery require you to develop the ability to accept the things you cannot change. Applying the Serenity Prayer (see exercise 6.7) and identifying the things you cannot change, as well as what you can do to better accept those things, will make noticeable, positive differences in your experience of pain and in your life. It is essential to remember that one thing you can always change is how you respond to the people, events, and situations in your life.

Applying the Serenity Prayer _____

{ *exercise* 6.7 }

Grant me the serenity to accept the things I cannot change, courage to change the things I can, and wisdom to know the difference.

Identify something related to your pain condition that you cannot change and need to accept.

_____

Describe how you will begin to go about accepting it.

_____
_____
_____

Identify something related to your pain condition that you can change.

_____

Describe how you will begin to go about changing it.

_____

_____

_____

Describe how you can tell the difference between what you can and cannot change.

_____

_____

_____

The following story provides a real-life example of the role that imbalances in thought can play in chronic pain and illustrates how the use of the techniques described in this chapter can help facilitate the pain-recovery process.

DAN'S STORY

I never expected that I would have to negotiate the challenges and complexities of chronic pain. As an experienced clinician with a master's degree, extensive training in psychotherapy, and an advanced credential in clinical hypnotherapy, I know a thing or two about the connections among thoughts, emotions, behaviors, and physical pain. However, with the onset of my own chronic pain condition in 1998, it was as if all my professional knowledge and experience disappeared.

After being diagnosed with herniated discs in my lower back, I allowed myself to become dependent upon conventional Western medicine with its reliance on opioid painkillers, lumbar epidural steroid injections, occasional episodes of physical therapy, and the ever-present option of spinal fusion. I effectively assumed the position of victim. In doing so, I submissively succumbed to the admonitions of my doctors (all extremely experienced, well-qualified, and well-intentioned) and relinquished sports and other physical activities that potentially put me at risk for further injury. As a lifelong athlete, this was an especially devastating loss. As I became more sedentary, I watched my physical functioning deteriorate further, as the vicious circle of chronic pain and addiction to medications prescribed for it progressively took over my world.

As a result of the mind-body connection, uncomfortable feelings and my inability to tolerate them created considerable stress, which only made my pain level worse — inviting, no, demanding that I use more and more narcotics. I began to feel increasingly helpless, fearful, depressed, and hopeless. This process unfolded over a period of eight years, gradually taking its toll on my family and career. In fact, my wife had been pleading with me to go into treatment for my dependence on the narcotic pain medication for several years. It reached a crisis point where I couldn't continue to live like I had been living.

Through a specialized pain-addiction program in Las Vegas, I received state-of-the-art education in the dynamics of pain and learned a range of alternative methods to manage my pain level. In treatment, I experienced a diverse array of holistic therapies including assisted stretching, massage, acupuncture, reiki, Chi Kung, yoga, targeted chiropractic, and physical therapy techniques I had never even heard of previously. Exposure to this comprehensive range of therapeutic modalities helped to significantly jump-start my healing process. Perhaps most importantly, I was empowered to become much more actively involved in the management of my chronic pain, and began to take ownership of it.

An essential part of my program of recovery is a daily morning self-care ritual that includes meditation, self-hypnosis, and nondenominational prayer, as well as stretching and Chi Kung exercises. Before treatment, my thinking usually fed irrational beliefs about my pain: "I shouldn't have pain," "This is intolerable!" "I have to take more pain meds," "Why me?" My overall level of stress is lower, which often has a positive impact on my coping capacity and functioning. I now maintain significantly different beliefs about my pain. I now often "talk back" to my chronic pain; not believing it and not buying into it. I still have pain regularly, but I deal with it very differently. It no longer debilitates me, dictates my activities, or controls my life.

In addition to my experiencing noticeably less suffering, my physical functioning has increased dramatically. I play tennis, bowl, and hike regularly, do strength training two to three times per week, and occasionally still play basketball. I maintain an awareness that, in return for participating in such activities, there will usually be some temporary increase in my pain level. I take the responsibility inherent in making a conscious decision to accept that trade-off.

In treatment I was introduced to a twelve-step program specific to my recovery from addiction to opioid painkillers. Working this twelve-step program has only strengthened my capacity to manage my chronic pain condition.

When I was a teenager and stuck in a negative, cynical mood, my father would tell me that "the city of happiness lies in the state of mind." At the time, I thought that was absolute bullspit. I know better now. I find that the more solution-focused I am, the more positive and hopeful I feel, and the less space my pain takes up in my head and in my life.

As of the time of this writing, I have not used any narcotic pain medications for over twenty-six months. Previously, I would not have believed this to be possible. My recovery process has given me the opportunity to rediscover interests and activities that were an important part of my life until pain and its prescribed course of treatment hijacked my brain, perverted my priorities, and sapped my spirit. Living with chronic pain isn't about waiting for the storm to pass ... it's about learning to dance in the rain!

Noticing Your Thoughts

Pain recovery includes working on consciously structuring your thought process to allow for acknowledgement and recognition of your thoughts without overreacting to them. Slowing down the thought process is the beginning of this process and will help you move toward balance. Instead of identifying your thoughts as indisputable facts, allow yourself to observe them with interest and curiosity. With practice, you will be able to witness your thoughts as they arise in your awareness.

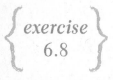

Slowing and Observing Thoughts _____

Take a few moments and observe your thoughts as they come up for you right now. Write three that come to mind.

_____

_____

_____

_____

Take a little time each day to practice these strategies to observe your thoughts and slow them down. We suggest you write about this daily in a separate journal or notebook.

As you can see from this chapter, the mind and the way we think affect every part of our lives. If we transmit distorted messages about reality, our experience will be out-of-balance. In the next chapter, we'll see that emotions are as significant of a factor in this process.

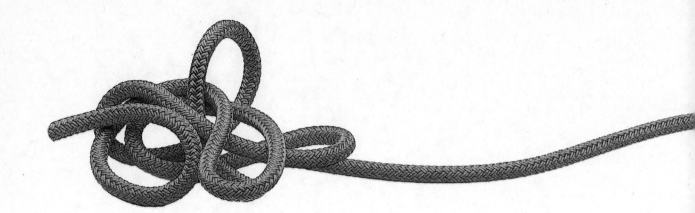

7

Emotional Balance

*A Cherokee elder was teaching his grandchildren about life. He said to them,
"A fight is going on inside me ... it is a terrible fight between two wolves.*

*"One wolf represents fear, anger, envy, sorrow, regret, greed, arrogance, self-pity,
guilt, resentment, inferiority, lies, false pride, and superiority.*

*The other stands for joy, peace, love, hope, sharing, serenity, humility, kindness,
benevolence, friendship, empathy, generosity, truth, compassion, and faith.*

This same fight is going on inside you, and inside every other person, too."

*They thought about it for a minute, and then one child asked his grandfather,
"Which wolf will win?"*

The old Cherokee simply replied, "The one you feed."

—author unknown

*Chronic pain includes both the physical experience of pain and the thoughts we have about it,
as well as the feelings associated with it. As we discussed in the previous chapter, the mind and
body share such intimate connections that they affect each other in direct and powerful ways.
Emotions are a critical part of the circuitry that links mind and body. This chapter will address
two essential questions:*

- *What is the relationship between chronic pain and emotions?*

- *How can this knowledge help you achieve emotional balance to cope more successfully
  with chronic pain?*

Emotional Extremes

Emotional extremes involve the significant imbalances of either feeling too much (overreacting) or too little (underreacting). Emotional imbalance includes not allowing yourself to experience your feelings as they evolve, suppressing or "stuffing" them, or being controlled by or "drowning" in them. Statements that reflect these respective extremes range from "I don't feel anything," "Nothing bothers me," or "I feel numb" to "I can't take it anymore!" "I just want to stop feeling this way!" or "I hate feeling this way!"

Underreacting is an extreme style of emotional responding that involves avoiding both feeling and expressing emotions as much as possible. This can happen unconsciously or as a result of conscious decision making. People with this emotional style rarely, if ever, seem to react with strong feelings. They keep their distance from emotions—they usually don't cry, and seem to treat virtually all situations as if nothing is a big deal. They learned early in life that expressing feelings is something to be avoided, and as a result, dealing with feelings directly—including actually feeling them at all—is unfamiliar, uncomfortable, and unsafe. Such individuals are much more comfortable in the realm of thoughts, thinking, and logic.

Overreacting is an extreme style of emotional responding on the opposite end of the spectrum. People with this style have minimal, if any, distance from the emotions they experience from moment to moment. They act out on their feelings immediately and impulsively and seem to be driven by emotions, with little or no thought or logic. They tend to react to most situations as if they are true crises, living in and constantly creating drama. The urgency and intensity of this drama can have the effect of pulling other people in like a whirlpool and involving them in the scenario. They don't just feel their feelings; they are consumed by them. Many people learned to overreact from growing up in environments where that style is prevalent, where emotions are expressed as soon as they are felt, without any conscious thought about the potential consequences of instantaneous, sometimes reckless venting.

Developing Awareness of Emotions

The capacity to identify, feel, and express emotions is essential to a balanced state. Yet many people have great difficulty identifying feelings and expressing them in ways that support emotional balance, especially in the presence of chronic pain.

There are several levels of awareness involved in cultivating emotional balance. The first level is becoming consciously aware that you are experiencing a feeling. Although you may not know specifically what the feeling is, it is important to simply notice and acknowledge that you have some feeling.

The next step is identifying what the particular feeling is. An important part of identifying your emotions is to put them into words. As an alternative to not knowing what you are feeling or feeling confused, it is helpful to *label* the feeling: "I feel anxious," or "I feel angry," or "I feel depressed." The more specific you can be in identifying your feelings, the more likely it is that you will understand the emotional experience.

Connecting Emotions to Bodily Sensations _____

{ exercise 7.1 }

Read through the list of feelings in the left column and circle the ones you are experiencing. Next, take a moment to think about them—it may be helpful to close your eyes and turn your focus inward—then, in the right column, indicate where you experience each feeling in your body. For example, anger might be felt as tightness in your shoulders, sadness as an aching in your chest, fear as a knot in your stomach, and joy as warmth in your heart.

Emotion	Where and How You Feel It in Your Body
Anger/Resentment	
Fear/Anxiety	
Grief/Loss	
Depression/Sadness	
Loneliness/Isolation	
Guilt/Shame/Embarrassment	
Ambivalence/Uncertainty	
Self-pity	
Serenity/Peace	
Love	
Hope	
Gratitude/Appreciation	
Compassion/Empathy	
Other: _____	

Learning how different emotions feel in your body in terms of their location (where you feel them) and sensation (what they feel like) will enable you to identify them more quickly and accurately.

Feelings Always Find a Path to Expression

Most people struggling with chronic pain and dependence on pain medication try to avoid emotional as well as physical pain. Our common thought process tells us that if we can just avoid the pain, it won't affect us. However, in the same way that lightning always finds a path to ground, feelings—including painful and uncomfortable ones—always find a path to expression. If we do not address and express them consciously and directly by allowing ourselves to feel them and talk about them, they will come out in indirect forms, often as unhealthy, self-defeating and/or explosive behavior. When feelings are expressed through behavior, they are typically operating unconsciously and outside our awareness and control.

That being the case, you have a choice in the way you deal with your emotional and physical pain. The choice is to address your feelings in the moment without further damaging yourself or others, or to avoid them and overreact in uncontrolled, dramatic ways. Allowing your painful feelings to be expressed through your behavior only adds more suffering to your life and the lives of others. Emotional balance gives you the capacity to choose which path you will take, instead of letting fear and avoidance make the choice for you.

Emotional Sensitivity

Another variable that can contribute to imbalance is emotional sensitivity. People who are emotionally sensitive feel things more rapidly and more deeply than others and tend to personalize them. Emotionally sensitive people may learn ways to numb themselves from their feelings because so many of their feelings are painful. For individuals with chronic pain in particular, feelings of anger, sadness, and depression are not only felt strongly, they are consuming, resulting in intensification of suffering and pain. Negative, uncomfortable emotions can become like a snowball rolling downhill. It gets bigger, gaining strength and speed as it continues. The longer it is allowed to roll without anyone attempting to halt its progress, the harder it is to slow it down or stop it.

You may use a range of strategies, including drugs and alcohol, to keep from feeling negative emotions. Pain medications, especially opioids, dull and distort the emotions. Drugs and/or alcohol actually increase emotional sensitivity whenever the acute effects of those substances—pain medications included—wear off. Use of mood-altering drugs for chronic pain can have substantial and adverse affects on your ability to identify, tolerate, and express emotions, creating imbalance in your emotional life. In pain recovery, you work to restore that balance. The rest of this chapter examines specific emotions that are normal and natural for everyone, but are especially relevant if you are dealing with chronic pain. These particular feelings result from and cause problems related to chronic pain and the effects of opioid pain medications.

Fear

With chronic pain, you may experience irrational and paralyzing fear. Irrational fear lacks reason and clarity. Paralyzing fear keeps you frozen in place, unable to move forward.

Fear is a natural human emotion that can help us to respond effectively to things that threaten us. Walking out into the middle of a busy highway appropriately causes fear. If someone points a gun at you and threatens to shoot you, obviously fear is a rational reaction to the situation. Fear becomes problematic when you allow it to debilitate you by keeping you from doing the things you need to do in order to function in the world. Also, it can be troublesome to be consumed by fear about something that *might* happen – anticipating the worst.

Taking pain medication can sometimes mask fear, making it easier to pretend it is not there. Fear feeds on itself; the more fearful you are, the more fearful you become, and the less able you are to function. Common fears associated with chronic pain are fear related to the pain itself; to doing anything that could possibly make the pain worse; to not having enough pain medication; to taking too much or becoming addicted to pain medication; to failed medical procedures or surgeries, loss of functioning or ability to do things; to job or career problems; to financial problems; to relationship problems; to getting worse or sometimes even to *getting better*; and the biggest fear of all, to getting off drugs. Many of these fears stem from fear of the unknown and/or fear of change.

Fear can be very difficult to acknowledge to yourself and others. Many of those who have lived with physical and emotional pain for a long period of time have learned to suppress their fear. Few people like to admit to or talk about being fearful. In some circles, feeling scared and expressing fear is viewed as weakness, making it even harder to discuss with others because of the desire to avoid negative perceptions and judgments.

It requires strength and courage to do anything that is uncomfortable or to do things differently from the way you've done them in the past. Therefore, rather than reflecting weakness, admitting to and talking about your fears reflects strength. Keep in mind that courage is not the absence of fear; courage is being aware of your fear and doing what you need to do in spite of it.

Learning about Your Fears _____

Identify your greatest fears as they relate to your chronic pain.

_____

_____

_____

_____

Describe specifically what it is about each of the above that creates fear for you.

_____

_____

_____

_____

Describe how living with these fears has affected your pain and your ability to get better.

_____

_____

_____

_____

_____

_____

Anxiety

Anxiety is a major cause of increased pain. Anxiety can be thought of as low-level fear. It can be defined as distressing uneasiness, nervousness, or worry felt in response to any situation you *anticipate* to be threatening. It is usually accompanied by self-doubt about your capacity to cope with it. Some of the physical symptoms of anxiety are sweaty palms, increased heart rate, muscle tension, breaking out in cold sweats, inability to sit still, and/or a feeling of being uncomfortable in your own skin.

A large percentage of people who have chronic pain report experiencing high levels of anxiety. They cite numerous reasons for this, including all of the issues linked to the fears commonly associated with chronic pain. It is common for people to take medications to alleviate fear and anxiety, in addition to the pain. The combination of imbalance, chronic pain, and medications is a fertile mix that anxiety thrives on.

An effective way to decrease anxiety is by learning and practicing relaxation and self-calming skills such as meditation, intentional deep breathing, progressive muscle relaxation, guided imagery, self-hypnosis, and even quiet downtime. Balanced individuals experience manageable levels of appropriate anxiety. A holistic approach will be most effective in helping you develop healthy habits to continue practicing in order to establish the emotional balance that will enhance your pain recovery.

Some things you can do to decrease anxiety:

- Reduce/limit caffeine consumption (definitely none after 4:00 pm).

- Pay attention to nutrition/limit sugar intake.

- Focus on the present/work on staying in the moment.

- Learn to meditate and practice diligently.

- Read recovery-related materials.

- Exercise as regularly as possible.

- Develop trust in the process of recovery to the best of your ability.

- Pay attention to spirituality—faith in something greater than yourself.

- Practice yoga.

- Practice Chi Kung.

- Explore reiki.

Taming Anxiety _____   { *exercise* 7·3 }

Identify the issues that bring up the most anxiety for you.

_____

_____

_____

_____

Describe how worrying about these issues is helpful to you.

_____

_____

_____

_____

How much time did you spend last week worrying about things that never happened?

_____

Identify at least three things from the list of suggestions given that you can begin to practice in order to reduce your anxiety.

_____

_____

_____

_____

Anger and Resentment

Anger is an emotional response to things that don't go the way we want them to. Anger results from the experience of feeling "wronged" in some way. Depending on the situation, anger is a healthy and appropriate emotional reaction. Problems with anger usually occur in how this powerful feeling is expressed. Anger can be expressed along a broad spectrum, from suppressing it (not expressing it outwardly) or keeping it inside to the point where you may not even be aware that you are angry, to exploding, such as with screaming, verbal abuse, or even physical violence. Anger and the resentment it can fuel can cause significant stress and high blood pressure, along with increased muscle tension and increased pain.

When you are in pain, you may unconsciously direct anger to the site of the physical pain ("My back is killing me!"). Anger might also be directed at yourself because you are unable to do the things you would like to do and/or were able to do previously. It may also be directed at others close to you, like family members and friends, for not understanding, not being supportive enough, or simply because they are in the wrong place at the wrong time. It is also common to be angry with the health care system, specifically the doctors who were unable to help you or who prescribed the medications that you became dependent on, or the insurance company that won't pay for the next procedure, let you see the next specialist, or pay for your disability. It is common to direct your anger at something or someone when you're really angry at something else. For example, you are angry because your back hurts, but you shout at your kids or kick the dog. This is referred to as displaced anger. Frequently, the more anger you have, the more it contributes to your level of pain, and the more out of emotional balance you are.

In most circumstances, anger is really a secondary emotion. It often forms immediately and automatically (this happens unconsciously, so there may be no awareness of it) in response to a situation that brings up feelings of hurt, fear, and/or inadequacy. Hurt and fear are the primary emotions that anger covers up. When most people experience these primary emotions, they feel vulnerable and their energy and attention are focused internally. This inward focus on one's own vulnerabilities is extremely uncomfortable, especially for individuals who are used to focusing on other people and things outside themselves. Anger serves several defensive purposes. It works as a shield that deflects uncomfortable primary emotions so they can be avoided or kept at a distance. Anger provides a sense of power and control, and directs focus outward to identifiable, external scapegoats. It is almost always easier and more comfortable to focus on the actions of others than it is to focus on yourself.

What can you do about anger? First and foremost, awareness that you are angry is necessary in order to make a conscious decision as to what to do about it. It is helpful to ascertain what you are really angry about—the true reason that you are angry. Knowing the source of the anger and looking beneath the apparent reason ("He's just a jerk") to a deeper level ("My feelings were hurt because he disappointed me") is valuable in examining your emotional reaction. The next steps in dealing with anger are identifying your wants and needs related to what's happening; selecting the solutions that are the best fit from the available options; and then taking action to implement those solutions. This solution-oriented process provides a direct route to finding balance and, consequently, turning down the volume on your pain.

*Looking More Deeply at Anger*_____

{ *exercise* 7·4 }

Describe the two most recent instances when you were angry.

_____

_____

Describe what happened to your pain level during these situations.

_____

_____

_____

_____

Now try to identify the underlying emotions in these situations that your anger may have been keeping under cover, such as hurt, fear, or inadequacy.

_____

_____

_____

_____

Be aware that you almost always play a part in the problems you experience. Identify how you may have contributed to the situation(s) that you were angry about.

_____

_____

_____

_____

_____

_____

Resentment is related to anger in that it is a negative feeling or ill will directed at someone or something experienced as wrong, unjust, insulting, or disrespectful. Anger is about the present, whereas resentment relates to the past. It is a reexperiencing of past events and the old feelings of anger connected to them. Resentment is created when we get angry at a person, institution, or situation, and hold onto that anger.

People can hold onto resentment for many years, refusing to let go, forgive, or forget, carrying their resentment wherever they go. Like an extra suitcase, it is baggage that weighs them down and requires attention and energy. Over time the person, place, thing, or event that caused the original anger and led to resentment may be forgotten, while the resentment remains like smoldering embers that are left after the flames of a fire have died down. The fire no longer rages, but the embers remain hot and capable of causing more fires in the future unless they are extinguished. As long as these embers continue to burn, they create negative distractions that take time, attention, and energy away from your pain recovery. As long as you are focused on the people and situations you are angry at and resentful toward, you are out of balance emotionally and typically feel more pain.

The continuous mental and emotional reenactment of past events that occurs with resentment reinforces feelings of being victimized. Feeling that you have been "wronged" makes you feel like a victim. This makes pain recovery more difficult because such perceptions interfere with the ability to take responsibility for your own choices and actions. The stronger the resentment is, the more time you spend thinking about it and caught up in the anger connected to it. This is a form of mental, emotional, and spiritual bondage. Ultimately, the person holding the resentment is the one who suffers most. After all, you can't change the past. So all you can do is shift your focus away from the past and toward being as successful as you can in the here and now.

The following are some techniques you can apply to deal with anger and resentment more effectively and regain emotional balance:

- Treat other people with fairness and compassion, even when you feel angry at or have resentment toward them. Notice what happens when you change how you act toward them in positive ways. They may change how they act with you.

- Practice expressing your anger and/or resentment in healthier, recovery-oriented ways: Talk about these feelings with *safe, appropriate* people; talk about them without yelling, screaming, threatening, or acting out; write about them; let go of them physically by working out, taking a run, going for a hike, or playing sports.

- Resist the urge to be a channel for the anger or resentment of others. The anger and resentment of others can be seductive — it can have an almost magnetic pull. Don't buy into it; resist the urge to join in their misery.

- Accept that the past is the past. It is as good as it's ever going to get! Give yourself reminders of this whenever you need to.

- Keep in mind that while anger and resentment are normal, natural emotions, you are always responsible for your actions. No one can "make" you do anything. You choose how you act and the choice you make is your responsibility. Acting out inappropriately can cause regret and further add to your anger and resentment.

- Stop expecting to be perfect.

- Notice what happens to your pain level whenever you apply these suggestions.

Letting Go of Resentment _____ { *exercise* 7·5 }

List the sources of your resentment.

_____

_____

_____

_____

Write a few ways to decrease their hold on you.

_____

_____

_____

_____

Depression, Sadness, Grief, and Loss

The feeling states of sadness, grief, and loss are closely related to one another and often fall underneath the umbrella of depression. Sadness refers to a feeling of unhappiness, while grief consists of distress related to the process of mourning a loss of some sort. Depression can be a feeling but is also a mood—a more enduring emotional condition that exists on a continuum. The most severe form of depression is a diagnosable disorder marked by a variety of symptoms that can include:

- Sadness.

- Difficulty sleeping or sleeping too much.

- Increased or decreased appetite.

- Weight loss or gain.

- Loss of interest and enthusiasm.

- Feelings of helplessness, hopelessness, and/or worthlessness.

- Decreased self-esteem.

- Fatigue or loss of energy.

- Poor concentration or indecision.

- Suicidal thoughts, thoughts of death, or suicide attempts.

Symptoms of depression frequently accompany chronic pain. When pain becomes a constant companion, you begin to suffer significant losses, including the ability to work and physically function as before, the ability to participate in previously enjoyed recreational and family activities, financial losses, and hopes and dreams for the future. Going through multiple medical procedures or treatments without noticeable benefit can add to feelings of depression. These losses characteristically lead to feelings of hopelessness, helplessness, and worthlessness. Depression is sometimes described as anger turned inward against oneself. If drug dependence or addiction to pain medication is added to the picture, the severity of these losses and the feelings that go with them typically increase, creating further emotional imbalances.

Unresolved grief can contribute to both pain and drug use. Grief is a natural state attached to loss. Loss occurs when someone or something is no longer available to us due to death, injury/illness or other health reasons, the end of a relationship, etc. The more emotionally important the loss, the greater the grief associated with it. Healing from grief involves mourning the loss and eventually accepting it. Mourning is a process of saying good-bye to and letting go of what you have lost. You may grieve the loss of your mobility, functioning, and old lifestyle because of your chronic pain. You may even grieve the loss of pain medications, which may have come to seem like your best friend, lover, and reliable confidant.

Acceptance of a significant loss does not mean that there is no longer any distress related to it. Losses that are fully accepted can still be painful, but they no longer create serious emotional imbalances which hinder health and healing. Much like a physical injury that has healed, there may always be a scar. Mourning and healing from grief is a process of regaining balance that takes time (months to years, generally) and is different for each individual. This healing process requires allowing yourself to fully feel all the uncomfortable, painful emotions that are part and parcel of saying good-bye to and letting go of people and things that were important in your life. Mood-altering medications themselves actually *cause* depression, though they seem to relieve it (only temporarily).

*Depression and Grief*_____

Identify any symptoms of depression you have experienced.

{ *exercise* 7.6 }

_____

_____

_____

_____

Describe two things you can do to help you through these symptoms of depression.

_____

_____

_____

_____

Identify your most significant losses, including losses due to chronic pain, and describe how you grieved each one.

_____

_____

_____

_____

Describe your understanding of what you need to do in order to more fully grieve and accept these losses and to heal and regain balance.

_____

_____

_____

_____

Loneliness and Isolation

Loneliness and the tendency to isolate oneself from other people are closely connected to depression, sadness, grief, and loss. However, this is such a fundamental issue for those struggling with chronic pain that we are addressing it separately. Loneliness is defined as a state of sadness due specifically to the emotional experience of being disconnected from others, of feeling and/or being, in reality, all alone. This feeling may come from a sense of being alone with your pain or alone with the disease of addiction, and believing that no one understands or can understand your situation. This experience can be so consuming that some have described it as feeling completely alone even in a crowd of people. Sometimes, the negativity you express is so severe that even those close to you may withdraw and keep their distance. And as with other emotions, pain sensations intensify.

Loneliness also is so often a problem for people with chronic pain because the onset of acute pain triggers an automatic response in most people to withdraw and "lick our wounds," a mechanism believed to have developed to help protect and preserve the species. It was, and at times still is, adaptive to isolate and rest when we are sick or in acute pain. Problems arise because chronic pain appears to stimulate this same desire to isolate, and ongoing long-term isolation ceases being adaptive and becomes a source of imbalance.

MARK'S STORY

For as long as I can remember, I felt an intense fear of being viewed as weak or negatively different from others. This fear was either caused or exacerbated by the fact that I was born with scoliosis, a relatively common hereditary disease that causes a curvature of the spine. When I was in fourth grade, I was told that I needed to wear a back brace to combat the progression of the curve. Being the only kid in a small school with an obvious illness was traumatic for me. Even though I was popular, relatively smart, and somewhat athletic, I felt ostracized by many kids because, in my mind, they thought I was limited in the things I could do or that I would be easily injured.

As time went on, I dealt with the problem by trying to ignore it. I would feign wearing the brace to sleep to please my parents, but by the time they came in to wake me up for school it was lying next to my bed. This worried them, but when they confronted me I reacted with manipulation. I would tell them that it restricted my breathing, that it was uncomfortable, and that they didn't understand because they didn't have to wear it. All of this was true, but it wasn't unbearable. I just hated the brace. I hated that it made me different, that it made me seem weak. I knew I wasn't weak, but I had to prove this to everyone else. So I started pushing myself— playing football, skateboarding, snowboarding, and doing dangerous things with my friends.

Ignoring the problem only made it worse. At the age of fourteen, I had a fairly extensive spinal fusion. Physically, I recovered quickly except for some noticeable weight loss, but emotionally, it would take me years. After the surgery I was essentially confined to my room for about four months. I went from about 130 pounds to 200 pounds and couldn't bathe because of the stitches, so, as you can imagine, I was a complete mess. During this time I felt completely isolated. I would hear stories about what other kids were doing and fantasize about how great it would be if I were there. Staying up all night and sleeping the majority of the day made me feel even more disconnected.

When I started high school, everything seemed to change. I began to have a social life. I wanted to be seen as the kid who was capable of doing everything, so I studied hard and I partied hard. Growing up in Las Vegas, the self-proclaimed City of Sin, it almost seemed like a badge of honor to be a drunk or an addict. I had to go to all the "coolest" parties because that was a reflection of my popularity and it would help quell the feeling of isolation that I had become so fearful of. When I started snowboarding again, I pushed myself so hard that I broke my collarbone on the first run. Later that year I broke it again. Living life in the fast lane began taking its toll, but because I was maintaining good grades and had gone through the surgery, I was able to dodge any real punishment from my parents and other authority figures.

When I moved to Portland, Oregon, for college, things changed again. College seemed to mimic the environment I lived in post-surgery. I was isolated, not knowing anyone, and stuck in a cold and dark place. Never seeing the sun—a fact of life in the Pacific Northwest—also took its toll. The rain and cold, coupled with the fact that I had broken a few more vertebrae and ruptured some more discs in my back while snowboarding, aggravated the day-to-day pain I felt. So I turned to my favorite crutch—drugs.

Because of my surgery, the majority of doctors I saw were more than happy to prescribe whatever pain meds I needed. My back was my drug cash cow, and I was going to milk it for all that it was worth. I began forging prescriptions and getting multiple doctors to write me numerous prescriptions at the same time. Eventually I began selling, which seemed to alleviate *the isolation I was feeling because everyone liked to be friends with the guy who had a constant supply of drugs and sold them cheap. It didn't matter that these relationships were completely superficial. To me, at that point in my life, these people were family.*

Eventually drugs, like they always seem to do, took me to an even darker place. I was put on probation at school because of possession of drugs, was almost shot, and generally lost all interest in life. At this point my parents became worried and I was sent to rehab after rehab, but either left or got kicked out of them. But eventually I took the first step, if only because all other prospects seemed so bleak.

Now clean for a year and not using pain medications to manage my chronic pain, I have found a new way of living. I have made deep personal connections with people and rebuilt those that I fractured during my insanity. I use other methods to manage physical pain such as stretching, keeping fit, remaining aware of situations that could aggravate my back, and when all else fails, distraction. When my back hurts I go to a meeting, read a book, or do anything that requires enough brain function to take my mind off the pain. I am able to snowboard now, as long as I take it easy. I play on a nationally competitive paintball team, which requires me to run, dive, jump, and crawl. I was also able to have an appendectomy that required pain medication and a general anesthetic without a problem, thanks to the tools and countless other people I have found in support groups that deal with those of us who seem to occupy a strange niche in the obscure diseases known as chronic pain and addiction.

{ *exercise* }
{ 7·7 }

Combating Isolation and Making Connections _____

Describe the ways you isolate from others.

_____

_____

_____

_____

List the people you feel most closely connected to.

_____

_____

_____

_____

Describe specific actions you can take to better connect with others, including both accepting and offering help.

_____

_____

_____

_____

Shame and Guilt

Guilt is an emotion wherein we feel that we've made a mistake. It is defined as a feeling of having committed some wrong or failed in an obligation. Shame, on the other hand, is an emotion where the feeling is that we *are* a mistake. Shame is defined as a painful feeling of humiliation or distress that may be caused by the conscious awareness of wrong or foolish behavior. Often it is not even attached to a specific behavior, but to how we perceive ourselves internally. These two feelings often exist in partnership for people with chronic pain.

The emotional experience of shame is based on a belief that there's something intrinsically wrong with you as a person. Deep inside you feel fundamentally flawed, and believe that everyone knows it. Having chronic pain feeds into and strengthens this belief. For many people, it is difficult to escape from the burden of shame that has been internalized as a result of growing up in families whose emotional style was to shower their members with shame through an ongoing torrent of put-downs, insults, and blaming. When you are "shame-based," anything you do that is less than exemplary reinforces the belief that you are defective and have been all along.

In addition to reinforcing shame, having chronic pain can be also be shame-inducing, along the lines of "I have this problem so there's obviously something wrong with *me*." This feeling can be further compounded by being dependent upon or addicted to pain medications because of the stigma attached to that. Shame is self-defeating to the point of being self-destructive.

Guilt is emotional distress or discomfort based on the belief that there is a problem related to your behavior, rather than to you as a person. It is ordinarily related to a specific action or an event. "Authentic" guilt can be healthy and helpful insofar as it's a sign that we've violated our own values or a more universal moral code. It helps keep us honest and self-aware in ways that contribute to emotional balance. In contrast, "false" guilt is a sense of responsibility for things that go wrong for which you are not responsible. It is easy to fall into a pattern of guilt-driven self-blame—for being in pain, for not being a "man" or "woman" anymore, for not being able to work or perform other physical activities as before; for not being able to stop taking drugs, etc. Feelings of shame and false guilt emerge when you begin to believe the lies that other people have told you about yourself.

The direct connection between thoughts and emotions is clear in patterns of guilt and shame that are enhanced by thinking characterized by shame-based statements, such as:

- ☻ I should be more patient with my spouse and kids; it's not their fault that I'm in pain.

- ☻ I should be back to work by now.

- ☻ I shouldn't be in this much pain.

Shame-based statements from others include:

- ☻ What's wrong with you?

- ☻ How could you do this to us?

- ☻ I wish we had never met.

{ *exercise* 7.8 }

Dealing with Shame and Guilt_____

Describe your strengths and positive qualities.

_____

_____

_____

_____

_____

Identify any lies that other people have told you about yourself that you can stop believing.

_____

_____

_____

_____

Describe how you can use the information above to achieve better emotional balance.

_____

_____

_____

_____

Self-pity

Self-pity is defined as excessive, self-absorbed unhappiness over one's own troubles. It is the emotional state of feeling sorry for yourself, sometimes in exaggerated ways. Self-pity is often a characteristic of chronic pain and addiction—after all, these troubles are very real. But the fact that self-pity often results from significant problems does not make it any less destructive in terms of its impact on emotional balance. When you are feeling self-pity, you are almost exclusively focused on what is wrong or not working in your life.

Practicing Gratitude/Focusing on the Positive _____

{ *exercise* 7·9 }

A solution-oriented way to regain balance when you're feeling sorry for yourself is to make a gratitude list. This can help you regain perspective and disrupt excessive focus on the negative.

Identify things in your life you are grateful for.

_____

_____

_____

_____

_____

_____

_____

_____

_____

_____

The Native American parable about the two wolves that battle for our hearts, minds, and spirits illustrates the importance of focusing on potential solutions as opposed to wallowing in problems, as well as how the choices we make play a central role in that process. Choosing to have conscious contact with positive feelings can help facilitate emotional balance.

{ exercise 7.10 }

Cultivating Positive States of Mind _____

Complete each of the following sentences with the first thing that comes to your mind.

For me, love means _____
_____.

My greatest source of happiness or joy is _____
_____.

It really touches my heart when _____
_____.

I feel most at peace when _____
_____.

I have the most compassion when _____
_____.

The person I feel closest to is _____
_____.

The things I appreciate most are _____
_____.

To me, faith refers to _____
_____.

I trust that _____
_____.

I feel grateful when _____
_____.

Sometimes you may think that you shouldn't feel the way you do. Feelings are neither good nor bad—they simply *are*. In the midst of intense negative feelings, whether fear, anger, depression, or whatever form they may take, it can feel as though they will last forever, like they will never end. It promotes emotional balance to maintain an awareness that all feelings are temporary, and that they will *always* change!

Emotional balance is achieved when you allow yourself to feel whatever comes up, and learn to accept your feelings without judging them. Because your feelings are a part of you, accepting them as they are is an important part of accepting yourself as you are. This is also known as self-acceptance. Whatever positive changes you want to make in your life, acceptance of how and where you are at the present moment is one of the keys to moving forward. Accepting your feelings also takes less energy than trying to avoid or suppress them, and helps maintain balance by eliminating the need for them to recur over and over. Genuine acceptance of your feelings gives you the opportunity to shift your energy to thoughts and actions that facilitate the learning, growing, and healing that can fuel the continuing progress of your pain recovery.

Our focus here is for you to learn and begin to practice strategies to identify and express emotions in ways that promote balance; deal with distressing, uncomfortable feelings in healthier ways; and strengthen positive feelings to promote growing, healing, and recovery from your chronic pain. For example, by finding enjoyable activities that you can still participate in and setting obtainable goals, you can shift your attention toward increased hopefulness, gratitude, potential solutions, and taking action.

Remember, your feelings can't hurt you, but reacting inappropriately to them can.

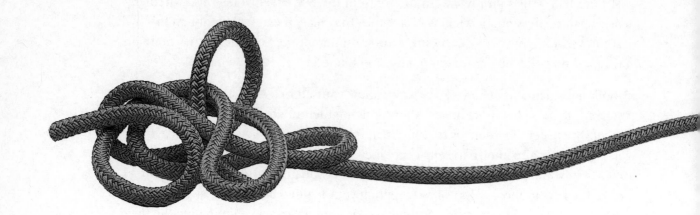

8

Spiritual Balance

In this chapter we will explore some of your basic spiritual beliefs and assist you in understanding the connection between spirituality and chronic pain. What exactly is spirituality? To start, let's consider spirituality as higher emotional functioning. By higher emotional functioning we mean concepts such as faith, hope, trust, belief, unconditional love, and a purposeful life.

- *Spirituality can be thought of as the area of life concerned with matters of the spirit, beyond oneself, though not necessarily in the religious sense.*

- *Spirituality includes a sense of connection to something greater than yourself, which may or may not include an emotional experience of religious awe and reverence.*

- *Spirituality includes a sense of connection to others, including emotional intimacy, and connection to the world around you — a feeling of belonging to a greater whole.*

When we talk about spirituality, it is important to note that we do not mean religion. However, spirituality does not preclude religion. For some, spirituality is closely connected to organized religion and a belief in God. For others, spirituality has absolutely nothing to do with organized religion and/or a belief in God. You can be an atheist and still live a spiritual life. You do not have to believe in a God to live a principle-centered life and believe in the inherent value of yourself and of humankind. The process of recovery allows you the freedom to choose what form your spirituality will take based on the right fit for you.

What Does Spirituality Have to Do with Pain or Addiction?

Living with chronic pain and addiction generally results in a lack of hope, faith, and trust. You can become so beaten down by the weight of your pain and dependence on opioids that your worldview becomes pessimistic, the majority of your thoughts center on various forms of doom and gloom, and your relationship to others and the world is increasingly negative. Faith, hope, and trust are fundamental components of the pain-recovery process.

Spirituality helps us reconnect with that which is greater than ourselves and our higher purpose. Spirituality broadens our horizons by lifting us out of a narrow, self-centered focus and helps us find meaning in our difficulties. If you think of pain or addiction as an affliction or a curse; if you think of yourself as a victim; if your mind frame is one of self-pity, your capacity to experience relief from chronic pain and stay clean will be greatly diminished.

Twelve-step fellowships have demonstrated, over many decades with millions of people, that the concept of coming to believe in a power greater than oneself is an essential part of the process of recovery. The same principle applies to pain recovery. This does not mean that you need to "believe" right now, but only that it will be helpful for you do the footwork and see what happens and what beliefs may come out of it. Spiritual beliefs are personal and individual, but we recommend you come to believe in a power greater than yourself that is loving, caring, and nonjudgmental, and only wants what is best for you.

Extremes of Spirituality

Most people would probably acknowledge that too little spirituality could be problematic, but is there such a thing as too much spirituality? In our view, yes—extremes in any of the points of balance will result in overall imbalance and interfere with the process of pain recovery.

One spiritual extreme is the rigid, insistent belief that there is nothing greater than the self, no purpose to existence or the universe, and certainly no God. This extreme frequently includes the perception that humankind is inherently "bad," and that people will always attempt to take advantage of you or get over on you if you don't keep your defenses up at all times. This extreme leads to fear, hopelessness, pessimism, distrust, and a sense that life has little or no meaning. Belief in nothing and/or no one beyond oneself swings the pendulum toward cynicism. It also tends to produce resentment toward those who are spiritual. From this perspective, those with spirituality are judged to be weak and dependent, and faith is equated with ignorance.

Another extreme is maintaining rigid, inflexible, "set-in-stone" beliefs that you have convinced yourself represent the absolute and only "truth." Most often, this attitude fuels a closed-mindedness that prohibits any actual examination of such beliefs and precludes openness to any other possibilities. This attitude is likely to occur when your concept of spirituality is based solely on religious dogma—positions concerning faith or morality formally stated and authoritatively proclaimed by a specific church or religion, without personal examination. At this end of the spectrum, all other beliefs, forms of spirituality, or conceptions of God typically have to be rejected as false or inferior since your belief is the one true way. In other words, because your belief system must be "right," all others have to be "wrong." This extreme position often breeds the intolerance for all other spiritual perspectives that goes hand-in-hand with religious zealotry. Intolerance is based on the inability to accept that there are alternative forms of spirituality with which your spirituality can peacefully coexist.

Another spiritual extreme is the belief that "God" will take care of everything, and you use this as a reason (or an excuse) *not* to take appropriate responsibility for making decisions and taking actions. When spirituality is seen as a cure-all for life's challenges, it can be used as a rationalization to avoid what you need to do in response to the circumstances life sets before you.

Spiritual Beliefs _____

{ *exercise* 8.1 }

Describe what spirituality means to you.

_____
_____
_____
_____
_____

Do you believe in God? If so, what is your concept of God? If not, why not?

_____
_____
_____
_____

Has your chronic pain and/or dependence on pain medication affected this belief? If so, how?

_____
_____
_____
_____

To what extent are you angry or resentful toward religion and/or God?

_____

_____

_____

_____

Do you have a clear picture in your mind of who you are and where you are headed in life?

_____

_____

_____

_____

_____

_____

_____

_____

Many Paths

Feeling confused or ambivalent about spirituality is understandable. The most important aspect of developing spirituality is being honest about your feelings, where you are at in your life, and what your beliefs are, along with how these beliefs manifest in your perspective, attitude, and behavior. Your challenge here is to be open to the possibility that growing a relationship with a power greater than yourself is a dynamic key to learning how to cope with life in ways that are balanced, healthy, and helpful.

There is no single path on a spiritual journey. In order to find the path that is right for you, you may travel many roads to get to where you need to go. On those roads will be many guides that will help you along the way. There is little to figure out or understand. There is no helpful purpose to be served in trying to find the answers; spirituality is not so much about answers as it is about learning how to appreciate the journey itself. The essence of spirituality is that it's an ongoing quest for meaning and fulfillment.

The parable of the two wolves also applies to your search for spirituality. Dependence on pain medications, isolating, resentment, fear, and anxiety have all fed your pain and contributed to imbalance. Here are some things you can do to feed your spirituality and move toward balance:

- Write about your thoughts, feelings, decisions, and experiences daily.

- Read materials that will help you on your path, present you with new information, and open new doors.

- Develop a mutual support system and attend support meetings regularly.

- Work the Twelve Steps and apply them in your life.

- Take care of yourself physically by staying active and exercising within your limits.

- Pray.

- Meditate.

- Share with others.

- Find ways to be of service, to help others.

- Stay present-centered in this moment; live just for today.

- Clear out old resentments and unresolved feelings so you can release these burdens.

- Laugh.

- Cry.

- Be grateful for what you have.

- Accept your pain and cherish the opportunities it provides you to grow and change.

- Make progress toward balancing the four points daily in order to change your experience of chronic pain.

There are no drawbacks to seeking a spiritual experience. You have nothing to lose and everything to gain. All that is required is for you to be open-minded and willing. On your journey, others may attempt to force their beliefs on you, but you are free to choose what you believe and do not believe. Try not to judge your experience or others' experience; just keep moving forward in your journey and notice what happens. There is more joy to be found in the journey than in any particular destination.

I cannot recall when my migraines started, but I do know I have had them for many years. I believe that I had about five years clean when I experienced my first migraine. I had to leave work because any light, sound, or other stimulation hurt so bad. I even found it difficult to drive myself to the doctor. At that appointment, the doctor told me I was having a migraine. He gave me some safe medication and had me lie down for a while. The pain seemed to let up enough so that I could go home and rest.

Throughout the years, the frequency and severity of my headaches has increased. I also experience different types of headaches, the migraines being the worst. There are times when my head literally feels like someone is cracking my skull from the inside, trying to get out. I experience nausea and sometimes throw up. The migraines wake me up at night, and there is nothing I can do but take Relpax or Imitrex and go back to bed. For the less severe migraines or stress headaches, I take ibuprofen, lie down for a bit, and then take a hot shower. By doing so, I can usually function well enough to work.

I can pretty much expect that a week before my menstrual cycle, I will have headaches that get worse and worse leading up to the first day. This isn't the only time I get really bad migraines, but it seems more likely to be when I will get the most debilitating migraines. Even if I can get the migraine to stop hurting so much, I am left with a feeling that reminds me of a hangover. I feel sick to my stomach and am unable to totally focus on work or whatever it is I am doing.

I have been clean for twenty-three years and I am grateful that, as of yet, the obsession to use because of the migraines hasn't been an issue. The most frustrating aspect of these headaches is that I miss out on my life when I am having them. I miss work, meetings, and get-togethers with sponsees, friends, and family.

When I experience any type of pain, my relief comes through prayer and focusing on taking care of myself by using safe medications and being able to live with a little discomfort. I know that the pain won't kill me, but if I use, I will surely die eventually. I have found that when I practice the Third and Eleventh Steps, I do gain strength from my loving God to get through the day.

Lack of Meaning in Life

Often the majority of meaning we ascribe to our lives relates to what we *do* and what we *have*. In other words, we tend to base the meaning in our lives on our careers and possessions. We commonly spend less time thinking about who we are on the inside and how that gives meaning and purpose to our lives. Material things can never fill internal voids. They may distract attention from internal emptiness or fill some of it temporarily, but such holes can only be filled from the inside. When we neglect who we are in favor of attending to what we do or what we have, our focus will always be outside of ourselves and we will miss the meaning of life because that meaning and purpose come from within.

Life Meaning

{ *exercise* 8.2 }

List three things you have (possessions) that contribute to your sense of who you are.

_____

_____

_____

Describe what makes these material things so important to your sense of self.

_____

_____

_____

_____

List three things you do (titles, roles, career) that contribute to who you are.

_____

_____

_____

Describe what makes these things so important to your sense of self.

_____

_____

_____

_____

_____

Taking a Spiritual Inventory _____

List five qualities that you consider positive and five qualities that you consider negative that contribute to who you are on the inside.

POSITIVE

_____

_____

_____

_____

_____

NEGATIVE

_____

_____

_____

_____

_____

Describe a minimum of three changes you can start to make to better balance your sense of self from the inside out.

_____

_____

_____

_____

_____

Intuition

An underrecognized facet of spirituality is intuition. Intuition refers to your inner voice that is always there. Being intuitive is similar to common sense, but with differences. Intuition means listening to your inner voice—not the voice in your head, but the voice deep in your heart that tells you if you are doing the right thing. It's usually a quiet voice that requires practice to hear. How many times have you said, "I had a feeling I shouldn't have done that," or "I should have followed my gut feelings?" Some of the variables that make hearing that voice more difficult are pain, medication, anger, resentment, and depression. By practicing pain recovery, you will intuitively make better choices based on what your inner self knows to be healthy for you. By practicing intuitiveness, you take responsibility for your spirituality without just relying on others to tell you what spirituality is or should look like.

Staying in the Moment/Living One Day at a Time

A number of approaches to spirituality emphasize the value of staying in the moment, that is, being present-centered in this moment, right here and right now, as opposed to focusing on what has already happened in the past or could potentially happen in the future. This also extends to the concept of living one day at a time. After all, you can neither change the past nor predict or control the future. The only aspect of time and experience that you have influence in is this moment and today.

There are many ways in which staying in the moment promotes health, healing, and pain recovery. In being present-centered and living just for today, you make yourself genuinely physically, mentally, emotionally, and spiritually available. Focusing on the past or on the future is an exercise in frustration and futility. Helpful techniques to stay in the moment and live just for today include concentrating on and deepening your breathing by paying attention to inhaling and exhaling; focusing on to five to ten things in the immediate environment, i.e., the room around you—walls, furniture, ceiling, etc.; and meditation and prayer.

Meditation and Prayer

Meditation is one of the essential components of living a spiritual life. Meditation quiets the chatter in our heads and allows us to gain perspective. You will find that practicing meditation will ease your physical pain and assist you in staying clean. The Eleventh Step in twelve-step fellowships talks about prayer and meditation in terms of using these practices as bridges to build a relationship with a power of one's own understanding that is greater than oneself. In this context, prayer is often thought of as a way to *talk to* one's source of spirituality, while meditation is a way to *listen to* that source of spirituality.

One form of meditation is based on mindfulness—that is, enhancing your conscious awareness of your internal experience. Sitting in a comfortable position with your eyes closed, let yourself relax and take note of body sensations, thoughts, and feelings. Notice them without judgment. Let your mind settle into the rhythm of your breathing. If your mind wanders (and it will), gently redirect your attention back to your breathing. Through meditation practice it is possible to face physical pain as well as uncomfortable and painful thoughts and feelings, and to learn simply to accept the pain or anger or sadness and let it pass without obsessing on or trying to change it. We strongly encourage you to find a meditative discipline that works for you.

Spiritual Principles

By acting in ways that are consistent with becoming aware of the wishes, feelings, and needs of others, and taking the needs of others into consideration when you make a conscious decision about how you want to act, you will experience greater balance spiritually and overall.

A solution-oriented strategy is to begin to develop a habit of thinking and acting consistent with the Serenity Prayer's guidance to "accept the things I cannot change," where you can accept your chronic pain as a part of your life and counteract it with the spiritual principle of surrender. Remember, paradoxically, surrendering to the things you cannot control or change is necessary to begin to reestablish the ability to choose how you want to act and what kind of life you want to have. One of the most important skills necessary to pain recovery is learning how to cope effectively with the often small but irritating normal and natural frustrations of life.

Maintaining the spirituality necessary for pain recovery can require ongoing practice in developing your understanding of and ability to apply such principles as patience, tolerance, acceptance, and humility. Patience is waiting without worrying and enduring without complaint. Tolerance is a spiritual principle that facilitates peaceful coexistence with physical pain and other feelings that are uncomfortable and/or painful, as well as with those people who may annoy, irritate, or otherwise upset you. Acceptance is about being okay with situations and people as they are, rather than focusing on how you want them to be or believe they should be. Humility is not thinking less of oneself, but thinking of oneself less.

The more that you can remain in conscious contact with these spiritual principles, the more balance you will have and the better equipped you will be to accept the full range of experiences that life will present you with.

{ *exercise* 8.4 }

*Finding Spiritual Balance*_____

Take a moment to list any extremes you are experiencing spiritually.

_____

_____

_____

_____

Describe what you think is needed for you to be balanced spiritually.

_____

_____

_____

_____

What, if anything, is holding you back from achieving this balance?

_____

_____

_____

_____

Another important part of the maintenance of pain recovery is cultivating an attitude of gratitude for whatever blessings you have. Sometimes you may have to look a little harder to see the blessings in your life, but there are always things to be grateful for, no matter how desperate the situation seems. You can learn, perhaps to your surprise, that it is possible to remain in conscious contact with gratitude in spite of feelings of physical pain, anger, depression, or fear.

The balancing effects of enhanced spirituality and its positive impact on your pain recovery may become apparent only gradually over time. It can be weeks or even months after these processes first begin before you realize that your awareness, feelings, and behavior have started to change.

When you build a balanced foundation of spirituality that is based on hope, trust, and faith, you maximize both your internal harmony and the potential for harmony between yourself and others.

RECOMMENDED READING

Everyday Tao: Living with Balance and Harmony, by Deng Ming-Dao; HarperCollins.

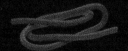

Part III

RECOVER

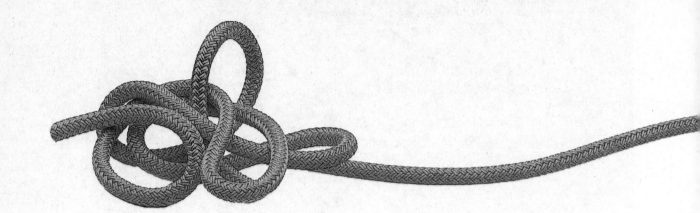

9

Relationships

There are numerous types of relationships, such as social, familial, intimate, romantic, acquaintance, and personal, all of which affect and are affected by your experience of chronic pain. Your relationships are not only an outward manifestation and an indicator of your overall state of balance; they also affect your state of balance either negatively or positively. This is why the relationships we choose are so important.

Living with chronic pain and/or addiction is guaranteed to result in relationship problems. While your tendency might be to jump right in and fix your relationships, we caution you that attempting quick fixes will only result in further imbalance. Resist the urge to work on your relationships, and keep the focus on yourself. As you work on your recovery, your relationships will become more balanced. The best way to resolve relationship issues is through slow, incremental changes based on your desire to achieve balance. Although it may sound selfish to you, now is the time for you to receive what you need.

Finding Mutual Support and Allies

Human beings are by nature social animals. As such, relationships with other people are of great importance to our overall well-being. In fact, research has demonstrated that social support is an important factor in determining how well someone with a chronic illness is likely to do in the future. Yet, as we've discussed, people who experience chronic pain with or without addiction are inclined to isolate themselves socially, effectively cutting themselves off from the balancing and health-enhancing effects of this social support. Research indicates that both loneliness and the pain that contributes to it are significantly lessened by a sense of connection with others, and the distraction offered by interaction with others. This is true whether or not the people who offer the distraction are known and loved by you. Telephone or Internet contact can also provide the double benefit of connection and distraction. Our approach to pain recovery includes seeking balance in this area through connecting with, accepting help from, and offering help to others as a way of life.

While some relationships are based on circumstances you have little or no control over, you do have choices in establishing relationships that provide support and nurture you. Twelve-step fellowships can offer you support and guidance from others who have found balance and are living in the solution. There you will find a sponsor, someone to guide you through the Twelve Steps and toward finding balance. You will also find role models and mentors to encourage and motivate you.

Participating in groups and fellowships such as these also helps complete the circle of giving and receiving by allowing you to give to others what was so freely given to you when it is appropriate.

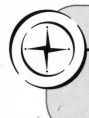

SUPPORT FOR FAMILY MEMBERS

Because chronic pain affects the entire family, finding mutual support and allies is also essential for the family of the person in chronic pain. Family members will benefit greatly if they enter a parallel recovery process.

RECEIVING

Accepting that you cannot deal with your chronic pain or addiction by yourself is essential to help you change old thought patterns and habits. You do not need to be or feel alone as you walk through this process. Living in isolation without the support and encouragement of others who truly understand will make recovery challenging. Friends, family, and others who are supportive of your recovery are helpful, but finding others who have experience with the new path you are on will provide the type of support you need rather than sympathy for your plight.

By building mutual support and allies, you will avail yourself of the personal and spiritual growth that comes from others sharing their experience, strength, and hope with you. Rather than viewing this as taking, look at it as receiving from others. Being able to receive requires admitting there are some things you can't and shouldn't attempt to do on your own. We strongly recommend that you ask for and accept assistance from those who have had a positive experience in areas with which you need help.

Allowing Yourself to Receive Help _____

How do you feel about others helping you?

_____
_____
_____
_____

What are your barriers to receiving help from others?

_____
_____
_____
_____

What can you do to overcome them?

_____
_____
_____
_____

Write about your experience with twelve-step fellowships or other group support. Were your experiences positive or negative? Why?

_____
_____
_____
_____

How can you integrate fellowship and supportive people into your pain recovery?

_____
_____
_____
_____

GIVING

After you have received what you need and are living in pain recovery, you will be ready to give back to others. Giving completes the circle of balanced relationships. But we must have something in order to give it. Many people think of giving back in terms of time, money, and resources. This is part of giving, but we are also referring to giving back our experience of how we achieved balance in our lives. Rather than giving advice, we share solutions and our experience, strength, and hope. We freely give to others what we have received, out of appreciation for what others have given us.

The ability to give back is a gift that recovery provides. When you get out of yourself, it helps you to see your problems in the proper perspective and context. It allows you to focus on things in your life for which you can be grateful.

{ *exercise* 9.2 }

Giving

Think about what it would be like if, two years from now, you are off all drugs, your pain is manageable, and you are balanced and content. Write about what you would share with others who are in the same situation as you were. How you would feel about sharing with them? What solutions would you share?

_____

_____

_____

_____

_____

_____

_____

WILLIAM'S STORY

In 1979 I was involved in a head-on collision that put me in the hospital for more than two weeks. My right leg was shattered in three places. I also suffered a ruptured spleen and was bleeding internally, so I had to be rushed into surgery to save my life. In a second surgery to repair my leg, I had to have an eight-inch plate inserted to hold the bone together so that it could heal properly. I woke up after that surgery with a cast on my leg that ran from my foot to my hip.

I remember lying in the hospital one night after surgery. The nurse had forgotten to properly replace the guardrail on my bed and my injured leg fell off the bed, causing me to scream. The nurse ran back into the room and gave me a pain shot. After that, I remember calling the nurse every four hours for my pain shot, even if I didn't need it, because of how good it made me feel. Before this experience, the only drugs I had used were pot and alcohol. I was released from the hospital and was prescribed pain pills, which I began abusing.

About two years after that accident I started to develop back pain, which became so severe I began to hunch over. It turned out I had a slipped disc that was pressing on my spinal cord and, once again, I had to have surgery. I was given a lot of drugs while in the hospital and several prescriptions for medications for when I was released. In the years that followed, I lived with self-destruction caused by my drug use and internal damage I still live with today.

In 1990 I went to a treatment center and found twelve-step recovery. I started attending meetings, got a sponsor, and began working the Twelve Steps. However, at the time I was unable to accept the principles, the traditions, and the steps because I had reservations. I held onto these reservations and they allowed me to justify my continued drug use for pain-related issues. I'd put my faith in doctors and I made them responsible for my recovery. I had legitimate physical problems and used those problems as an excuse to take pain pills. The self-pity that I felt was enormous. This was a common theme of my existence for about ten years, and in that time I joined and left my twelve-step program many times.

Pale gray, with abscesses on my arms and ready to die, I surrendered. I got a sponsor and went into treatment. That was my last time in a treatment center. Deep inside me, a change happened. I no longer wanted to continue using. I spent five days in the treatment center detoxing off heroin, pain pills, antidepressants—and self-pity. When released, I went to a meeting that night and every night for eighty-seven of the ninety days following treatment. For the first three weeks after treatment, I felt like I was going to die. I even went to a twenty-four-hour convenience store to buy an alcoholic beverage, but they didn't sell alcohol. I then drove across the street to a grocery store and just sat in my car for a while. I said "Okay, God," and drove home.

I now have over five years clean, and I live with chronic pain. I have learned that I can live with chronic pain no matter how hard it may seem because today I have a complete desire not to put drugs into my body. I have learned to live a normal life with very few limitations and to be happy.

For addicts who have pain, this is not possible, in my opinion, without the Twelve Steps, the use of a sponsor, attendance at meetings, the help of other people, and a loving Higher Power that I choose to call God. In addition to these resources, I must possess the desire to change into what God wants me to be. To achieve my God-given potential, I must be able to help others. This is but one of the principles that I have found in my twelve-step program.

It is true that all addicts suffer from emotional pain and physical pain in the beginning of their recovery; however, not all addicts continue to live with physical pain. Those of us with chronic pain need a place where others understand the pain we live with. I have been given the opportunity and the courage to begin attending the Pain in Recovery Support Group (PIRSG). I know that not all people who suffer from chronic pain are addicts, and I welcome nonaddicts and those with chronic pain to share in my recovery as I share in theirs. We share a common bond — chronic pain — and together we can learn to live free.

I am free from active addiction and experience the relief from having to use drugs to live with chronic pain. By working the Twelve Steps, I have found that anything is possible. The only limits to my recovery from addiction and chronic pain exist in my head.

WEB RESOURCE

Pain in Recovery Support Group (PIRSG): www.paininrecovery.org

Relationship Patterns

Relationship patterns are established early in life. Our parents, role models, friends, etc., influence how we view ourselves and others and have an emotional impact throughout our lives. For example, the way you treat others is influenced by the way your parents acted toward each other. If we never examine these patterns we tend to repeat them, no matter how unhealthy they are. You can probably identify several examples in others' lives where you observe repeated dysfunctional behaviors, and you wonder why they keep happening. Identifying your own patterns is a significant step in helping you to choose relationships where you support others and they support you in a mutually beneficial give-and-take.

The depth and quality of your recovery is enhanced
by the depth and quality of your relationships.

{ *exercise* 9.3 }   **Relationship Patterns**_____

Write about patterns you learned early in life that affect your relationships today.

_____

_____

_____

_____

_____

_____

Reviewing Your Current Relationships

It is important to take inventory of your current relationships so you can identify those that will help or hinder your quest for balance. We encourage you to assess your current relationships and alter or let go of unhealthy associations and focus on healthy relationships with people who are sincerely interested in your well-being.

Assessing Relationships _____

{ *exercise* 9·4 }

Make a list of all the significant relationships in your life.

◉ _____   ◉ _____

◉ _____   ◉ _____

◉ _____   ◉ _____

◉ _____   ◉ _____

◉ _____   ◉ _____

◉ _____   ◉ _____

Now review your list and place each relationship into the following categories.

BALANCED AND SUPPORTIVE   **IMBALANCED AND DETRIMENTAL**

◉ _____   ◉ _____

◉ _____   ◉ _____

◉ _____   ◉ _____

◉ _____   ◉ _____

◉ _____   ◉ _____

◉ _____   ◉ _____

If you were able to choose someone to assist you in your pain recovery, what would he or she be like and why?

_____

_____

_____

_____

_____

_____

Other Relationship Dynamics

SICK ROLE

When someone in the family has chronic pain, family roles and responsibilities often change, with the chronic pain sufferer taking on a more dependent status, or "sick role." The spouse or partner of the person in pain may start to take on too many responsibilities. He or she may feel more like a nurse or parent than a partner. This role shift can lead to feelings of resentment and frustration. The increased stress on the relationship often leads to arguing or conflict, as well as isolation, withdrawal, and even estrangement.

This is especially problematic if you have good days with your pain, where you can function nearly normally, and bad days, where you can't function well or feel like doing very little. This pattern can create uncertainty and confusion. Unlike acute pain, which has an end point, chronic pain goes on and on, increasing frustration in the family.

Since you are not getting better and there is no indication of if or when you will be able to resume your usual healthy roles, everyone's roles and expectations become murky. Knowing this seldom makes the strain, uncertainty, or resentment any easier to deal with. Family, friends, and coworkers end up feeling as controlled by the chronic pain as you do, and what's tough about that is that they don't have any socially sanctioned way to deal with their feelings. They may be afraid that if they talk about their feelings, they will be perceived as complaining or as a "whiner."

When the strain of trying to cover more responsibilities is added to this conflict, your loved ones' suffering can be quite profound. Their suffering is increased by the unpredictable nature of chronic pain—their not being able to predict on any given day (or hour) how good or bad you will be feeling. By recognizing the impact of your pain on those around you and communicating clearly when you are feeling better or worse, without demanding attention or sympathy, you can help ease the pressure on your loved ones. In short, don't overstate your case, but don't leave them guessing. There are times when their pain, though not physical, is as great as yours. In fact, brain studies have shown that some people, when observing another person in pain, show increased brain activity in the same regions as the person in pain. In other words, they truly "feel your pain."

It is also not uncommon for family members to experience secondary gain from your illness. They adapt to your sick role and may even be uncomfortable as you improve, because the equilibrium is shifting yet again. In the extreme situation, their identity has become that of caregiver, so if you get well, they may lose their sense of purpose and direction. This dynamic makes it all the more important for families to receive help as you proceed through pain recovery.

CODEPENDENT BEHAVIOR AND RELATIONSHIPS

Most people have heard the term "codependence." Codependence originally referred to an addict being dependent on drugs, and the partner in the relationship being dependent on the addict, and thus codependent. However, codependency is not just a characteristic of addiction. Dependent behavior is exhibited in many relationship dynamics. For individuals with dependent tendencies, being in a relationship that requires taking care of someone (e.g., a person with chronic pain) is a perfect scenario for these tendencies to flourish. Typically, a codependent person feels compelled to meet the needs of other people, and to fix or control others. As a result, the codependent person unknowingly enables and contributes to his or her partner's continued imbalance (addiction, chronic pain, etc.). For example, your spouse, partner, or someone else close to you may enable your isolation and withdrawal from the family by not confronting you or not communicating how upsetting it is. There is a study showing that in the presence of a "solicitous spouse" (one who genuinely cares and expresses concern), your pain increases.

It should be noted that this discussion of codependence barely scratches the surface of an important and complicated topic. Many good sources of information on codependence are available, and we recommend further reading on this topic.

Identifying Codependency in Self and Others _____ { *exercise* } 9.5

This exercise will help you to identify dependent traits in yourself and in someone with whom you have a close relationship (this can be a spouse, romantic partner, or other significant relationship). Read the following list of characteristics and indicate which apply to you, to the other person, or to both of you (check both boxes).

Self	Other Person	Characteristic
		Problems trusting others (anticipating betrayal), making true intimacy very difficult.
		"People-pleasing," an excessive need or desire to do what other people want, often at the expense of one's own needs.
		Covering or making excuses for behavior so as to avoid having to deal with the consequences (e.g., telling family that someone is "sick" or "tired" when he or she has taken too much pain medication or is drunk).
		A need to be in control of self and others at all times.
		An excessive need for another person's approval or guidance.
		Discounting or doubting one's own judgment—always being worried about making the wrong decision.
		Always ending up in relationships with people who need to be taken care of.
		Always ending up in relationships with people who initially need help, but later take advantage or become abusive in some way.
		Fear of feeling angry (i.e., losing control), to the point of avoiding confrontation or conflict and/or denying that one is angry.
		Lying, omitting information, or exaggerating, even when it would be easier to tell the truth.
		Fearing abandonment—would rather be mistreated or abused than be alone.

Finding balance in life requires that we interact with the world, specifically other people. Healthy relationships, which involve giving and receiving, are an essential part of pain recovery. These relationships will allow you to accept help from others and, by reaching out, will enable you to get out of yourself and leave the burden of your suffering behind.

RECOMMENDED READING:

Choicemaking: For Spirituality Seekers, Co-Dependents and Adult Children by Sharon Wegscheider-Cruse; Health Communications, Inc.

Adult Children: The Secrets of Dysfunctional Families by John & Linda Friel; Health Communications, Inc.

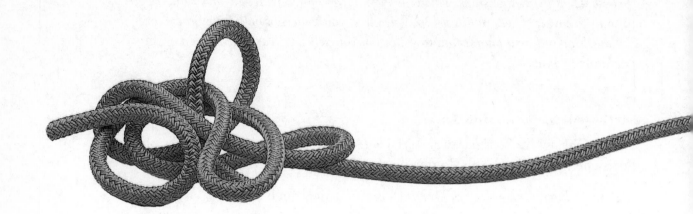

10

Positive Action

Now that you understand the four points — the essence of who you are — and the kinds of impact they have on your relationships and the world, let's look at how your state of balance will manifest in your life — in other words, your actions and behaviors. Most of us try to "think our way into good action." Twelve-step recovery recommends that you "act your way into good thinking." We will adapt this concept to pain recovery and apply it to each point.

You will be ready for this chapter when you have taken a leap of faith, removed pain medications from your life, and are living in pain recovery. No one who is actively practicing the principles of pain recovery will relapse. Relapse, in the addiction literature, refers to returning to drug use and an unhealthy lifestyle. In pain recovery we refer to relapse as it relates to drug use, as well as to a return to a state of imbalance due to losing track of the healthy changes that you have been able to implement in your life.

When we relapse, we lose sight of the advantages of recovery and look for short-term, immediate gratification. To be in pain recovery means to be in balance. This includes full acceptance of the problem and fully implementing the solution in all areas of your life. When you have found balance in body, mind, emotions, and spirit, relapse prevention is better labeled recovery maintenance and enhancement, which deals with the positive, not the negative. Pain-recovery maintenance involves continuously monitoring each point and your overall experience, actions, and relationships to stay in balance.

Imbalance usually results from not practicing what we've learned in pain recovery. Be careful not to judge yourself for letting up on your recovery — none of us do this perfectly or are always correct and consistent. You simply need to recognize the signs of relapse and become adept at identifying them as early as possible. Then you can take an action to correct a particular point, get back in balance, and resume recovery. Here, positive action is the key.

Let's look at how each point can become unbalanced and may cause us problems. These are things to watch out for. For each point, we will ask you to create an action plan to return to a balanced state.

Imbalance of Physical Life

Imbalance of the body can manifest as fatigue, aching, nausea, sleep disturbance, and increased pain. Medication use affects your body. Stopping opioid medications under medical supervision (medically-managed withdrawal) will cause a physical upheaval for a time, and balance may be difficult to achieve until your body recovers its own store of endorphins. It is important to work on balance during this time to offset the physical discomfort that is part of withdrawal. During these times it is crucial to get support in the other points, including thoughts, emotions, and spirituality.

Maintaining balance in your physical life entails continuous monitoring, but not judgment, about your state of nutrition, energy, exercise patterns, and ingestion of toxins. It also involves taking care to avoid extremes. If you exercise excessively, you may burn out and stop exercising completely. If your diet is healthy but too strict, you are likely to eventually overindulge and return to unhealthy eating habits. Maintaining physical balance involves monitoring your body as well as emotions associated with your body. Of course, the level and nature of your physical pain plays a big part in becoming imbalanced physically.

{ *exercise* 10.1 }

*Creating an Action Plan for Physical Balance*_____

Describe what happens when you feel tired.

_____
_____
_____
_____

Describe what happens when your pain is bad.

_____
_____
_____
_____

Describe what happens when you can't sleep well because of your pain.

_____

_____

_____

_____

What are some other physical issues that make you feel imbalanced?

_____

_____

_____

_____

ACTION PLAN

When I am tired, I will take the following actions:

_____

_____

_____

_____

When I am in more pain, I will take the following actions:

_____

_____

_____

_____

When I can't sleep, I will take the following actions:

_____

_____

_____

_____

When I have other physical problems, I will take the following actions:

_____

_____

_____

_____

As I am coming off medications, I will take the following actions to support myself through the physical symptoms:

_____

_____

_____

_____

Here is a series of physical actions I'm committed to taking on a regular basis:

_____

_____

_____

_____

_____

_____

_____

Imbalance of Thoughts

The experience of pain will often set off unbalanced mental functions. When you find yourself hurting, your thoughts become distorted again and you may think of taking an opioid medication to relieve the pain. You might tell yourself, "I have pain and the drugs are the only thing that will help take the pain away." During these times, it is easy to forget all the additional pain and confusion that the drugs caused and how you ended up being controlled by both the pain and the drugs. When your thoughts are imbalanced, they may tell you that it will be different this time or that you will be able to remain in control.

This type of thinking may lead to trying to find easy ways out of situations, like seeking immediate relief, without seeing that there are other, often better, options available. You may forget all the things that have worked to relieve your pain *other* than drugs.

If you forget that you are in control of your life and return to feeling like a victim of chronic pain, you may find yourself asking, "Why me?" Freedom from victim-thinking is realizing that "Why not me?" makes much more sense. It can be helpful to remind yourself that you are one of millions who have the same problems or worse.

Be mindful of the messages you are telling yourself. Negative self-talk about the futility of any effort, feeling sorry for yourself, and believing that others really don't understand what you're going through are manifestations of being out of balance. Feeling unique and different will make you less likely to look to others for help or have any interest in helping someone else, leaving you out of balance and in dangerous territory.

Of course, how you think influences how you feel, which affects your actions. It is difficult if not impossible to have irrational thoughts and not act out with irrational behaviors.

Creating an Action Plan for Mental Balance _____

{ *exercise*
10.2 }

How did you convince yourself in the past to stay on your pain medications?

_____

_____

_____

_____

_____

_____

How might you justify taking pain medications after being off them again?

_____

_____

_____

_____

What other thoughts come up that get you out of balance (e.g., black-and-white thinking, making things worse than they are, etc.)?

_____

_____

_____

_____

ACTION PLAN

List what actions you need to take when each of the negative thoughts you listed, about taking medication or other issues, comes up:

_____

_____

_____

_____

_____

_____

Imbalance of Emotions

It is common in life, especially if you have chronic pain, to experience challenging situations that provoke negative emotions. Our responses are difficult, though not impossible, to change. We have already described the nature of using pain medications to treat both physical and emotional pain. Without the medications on board, you may experience emotional imbalance in the form of fears (rational and irrational), anger, anxiety, sadness, and frustration. You may also find yourself feeling excitement, happiness, and even elation. These feelings may come up in ways you're not used to dealing with; it is the challenge of dealing with emotions in an appropriate, healthy manner that finding balance will provide.

Having feelings and not being aware of them is another aspect of emotional imbalance. Unless you know what you are feeling, you may fall victim to these feelings and be powerless to control them.

It takes hard work to change these patterns, the kind of work you have done so far. But to sustain the changes, continuous vigilance about your emotional responses to circumstances that arise in your life will be required.

{ _exercise_
10.3 }

_Creating an Action Plan for Emotional Balance_____

Emotions may arise when we are not aware or paying attention. Take some quiet time and write about what it's like to:

Feel angry or frustrated with pain or life circumstances.

_____

_____

_____

_____

Feel afraid or uncertain about pain or life circumstances.

_____

_____

_____

_____

Feel lonely or sad about pain or life circumstances.

_____

_____

_____

_____

Feel happy and successful about pain or life circumstances.

_____

_____

_____

_____

ACTION PLAN

What actions you will take when you have negative emotions?

_____

_____

_____

_____

_____

Imbalance of Spirituality

Since spirituality is so individualized, the ways we get out of balance are unique. Some patterns to watch out for include losing a sense of God or Higher Power and not praying, meditating, or using other spiritual practices. Becoming self-reliant, isolated, and self-consumed may lead to engaging in unhealthy behaviors.

Conversely, becoming overzealous and neglecting family, work, friends, and other activities for spiritual practice is another form of imbalance to watch out for.

As your nervous system "wakes up" without pain medications, you are likely to think, feel, and have bodily experiences (namely, pain) that throw you off balance. If you are unable to get past the experience in your mind and body to find a greater, expanded version of your existence, it may drag you down and keep you stuck in your "defective" self.

{ *exercise* 10.4 }

Creating an Action Plan for Spiritual Balance _____

How have you become removed from your spiritual "comfort zone" in the past?

_____
_____
_____
_____

Describe challenges for which you can allow for a power greater than yourself in your life.

_____
_____
_____
_____

ACTION PLAN

List the actions that bring you closer to your spiritual self and that you will maintain to stay in spiritual balance.

_____
_____
_____
_____
_____
_____

BEN'S STORY

I've heard a lot of stories about people using mood-altering substances to help alleviate physical pain and ending up addicted. My story is one of finding recovery and, after being clean for a couple years, experiencing more physical pain than ever before. I hope my story helps someone know they're not alone.

The Emotional Pain of Active Addiction

From the age of sixteen, I have experienced lower back pain. It usually came and went and was more aggravating than anything else. Around the age of twenty, after my father died, I started using various substances on a regular basis in an effort to mask the emotional pain I felt. Social use quickly spiraled into active addiction.

After seven years of fighting with the disease of addiction and losing, I finally surrendered. Getting and staying clean has brought (and continues to bring) a lot of joy to my life. When I got clean I didn't have much, but I was grateful for what I did have. I once again became employable, so I got a job in a field I had some experience with: cabinet making.

And Then There Was Physical Pain, Lots of Physical Pain

Construction work of any kind can be hard on a person's body, and I was no exception. Periodically I would experience lower back pain, but it would usually pass after a few days of rest. Looking back, I can see how the periods of pain increased over time. I never went to a doctor or pursued any medical help. Instead I would just tough it out. Then, at about two years clean, I experienced the worst pain I had ever felt up to that point. My back had been hurting for weeks and I was having trouble walking, much less working. My employer also had back pain, so he took me to his chiropractor's office. At that point I was willing to do just about anything to stop the torment. I had shooting pains going down my leg, and it literally felt like someone was constantly stabbing me in the back. I tried a few chiropractors before finding someone I trusted and who actually gave me some relief. The adjustments began helping so I continued to go. I was making progress.

The Setback

One morning I woke up and attempted to get up when the pain hit, and I do mean hit! I wasn't able to stand up, and my foot was going numb. I was completely freaked out, so I called my wife. She immediately called our friend, a nurse practitioner, who advised me to go to the emergency room. My mother-in-law arrived a few minutes later to give me a ride, and off to the hospital we went.

After a medical student examined me, I told him that I was an addict, so under no circumstances did I want any type of narcotics prescribed. This clearly baffled the young man. He left, and a few minutes later a resident entered and requested more information about the substances I was addicted to. It appeared they were confused because I had never used opioids before; they understood addiction only as it related to specific substances and couldn't understand why I was taking such a strong position against taking pain medication. Next, the attending physician came in. She assured me that she was well-informed about the disease of addiction and then proceeded to offer me muscle relaxers as an alternative to opioids. I couldn't believe what I was hearing. I was doing my best to be responsible for my recovery by explaining that I didn't want any type of medications that would work on that part of my brain. I wanted to know what I could do to address the pain, not what I could do to mask the pain. My disease started doing back flips inside my head, telling me that taking muscle relaxers or some kind of pill was justified. I had been in pain for months now, and the thought of some relief was tempting, but the recovering part of me won out and I declined the prescription. The doctor said there was really nothing else that could be done for me, and that I should set up an appointment with my regular doctor.

I spent the next several months going to the chiropractor several days a week, sometimes two or three times a day. I would get somewhat better, then have a setback—a pattern that went on for months.

An Eye-Opening Experience

During one of my setbacks, I remember calling my sponsor to give him one of my "woe is me" stories. After listening, he asked if I was doing exactly what the doctors had been telling me to do. I paused, and said that I was, for the most part. He wanted to know which recommendations I wasn't following, and I admitted that I had been lifting and twisting a lot at work, engaging in the very activities and movements that my doctor had advised against. I had convinced myself that I would be fine, that the lifting and twisting weren't part of the problem. Then, my sponsor said something I'll never forget. He said, "Who's to say that this isn't your disease convincing you to do things that will hurt, knowing that it will keep you stuck in your pain and make using more appealing?" My stomach flip-flopped. In recovery I've learned to pay attention when my stomach behaves like that, because it's telling me to listen up. He reminded me that if I wanted something different, then I needed to do something different, and that he cared.

Progress, not Perfection

Since that point I've changed my activities at work, and my back has consistently gotten better. I finally learned that the source of the pain is a bulging disc in my lower back that pinches *nerves on both sides of my spine. I've been given multiple nerve-block injections in my back. I continue to see a chiropractor at least once a week and I've also gone to an acupuncturist a few times. I exercise on a regular basis, with my doctor's approval, which helps break up the built-up scar tissue around the disc and strengthens the muscles that hold my spine in alignment. I no longer smoke, so my circulation and overall health have greatly improved.*

To take care of myself emotionally and spiritually, I talk about my physical pain with my sponsor, support group, and Higher Power. I attend twelve-step meetings, standing up at the back of the room if the pain is too great to sit. I also do my best to apply the Twelve Steps in my approach to pain. There are things that I can control, like how I treat my body, and things that I can't control, that I need to turn over to my Higher Power and then have faith that as long as I do what I'm supposed to, all will be well. Most mornings I experience pain, usually about a two or three on a scale from one to ten. Instead of lying around focusing on the pain, I get up, read my meditation, pray, and then begin my day with a healthy meal. This is my way of doing something different: participating in recovery and the solution.

Connecting the Points of Balance

THE RELATIONSHIP BETWEEN THOUGHTS AND EMOTIONS

A common misconception is that emotions or feelings occur in direct response to a sensory event. Such events can be internal, such as our physical state (e.g., a backache), or external to us (e.g., being stuck in traffic). So it may seem that the event causes the resulting emotion. Yet, in response to an event, thoughts actually occur before feelings. It is the way we think about the event, our beliefs about it and how we interpret it, that creates our emotional response. Our emotional response, the way we feel about an event, then, has great influence over our consequent actions.

This helps explain how different people can experience basically the same event and have completely different feelings in response to it. For example, two women are waiting to be picked up by their husbands after work. They were expecting to be picked up at 5:00 pm and it is now 5:20. The automatic thoughts that occur to the first woman go something like: "He's so late. He obviously doesn't care about me enough to get here on time!" In contrast, the thoughts that come up for the second woman are: "He's so late. Traffic must be especially heavy." Based on those different thoughts, and the divergent beliefs about the same situation that those thoughts represent, the emotions each of these women feels are likely to be very different. Place yourself in each position for a moment, thinking each of those different thoughts. What feelings come up for you in response to each set of thoughts?

In response to this same event, there are multiple different thoughts that could occur automatically, including, but not limited to: "He must have forgotten about picking me up"; "I wonder if everything's okay"; "Maybe the kids' practice ran late"; "I hope he didn't get into an accident." Each of these thought responses has different beliefs or interpretations attached to it, and, in turn, each belief or interpretation is likely to generate different feelings in response to the same event.

{ *exercise*
10.5 }

Connecting Thoughts and Emotions _____

Describe an event you have experienced where the initial thoughts you had and your beliefs about the situation turned out to be inaccurate.

_____

_____

_____

_____

_____

Identify the feelings that came up for you in response to your thoughts about this event.

_____

_____

_____

_____

_____

Imagine yourself back in the situation and change your initial thoughts and beliefs so that they match what actually happened. Identify the feelings that come up for you now in response to these changes in your thoughts and beliefs about the event.

_____

_____

_____

_____

Notice how different the feelings that came up for you were after you changed your initial thoughts and beliefs to accurately fit the situation, compared to your first set of feelings.

HOW DOES THIS PROCESS RELATE TO CHRONIC PAIN?

If, in our example, it were you waiting to be picked up by your spouse or a friend after work and you have a chronic pain condition, and your automatic thoughts and the beliefs related to the event are negative (e.g., "He doesn't care enough about me to get here on time"), the emotions that result are frustration and/or anger. Frustration and anger lead to increased muscle tension and stress, which generally lead to increased sensations of pain.

There is a correlation between negative thinking and beliefs and the level of pain you experience—the more negative the thoughts and beliefs, the greater the pain sensations. This can quickly become a vicious cycle as pain triggers negative thoughts and self-talk that can then translate into suffering, as well as increased muscle tension and stress, which, in turn, amplify the pain signals, triggering more of them. The longer such a cycle continues, the more out of balance you may become.

The progression is essentially as follows:

Event (overshadowed by chronic pain)

⬇

Negative thoughts/self-talk/beliefs

⬇

Suffering/anger/depression/fear/anxiety

⬇

Muscle tension and stress

⬇

More pain

⬇

Increased negative thoughts/self-talk/beliefs

⬇

Greater suffering

The process of pain recovery includes dramatically changing this negative progression through regaining balance in thinking.

Reestablishing balance counteracts this negative progression thus:

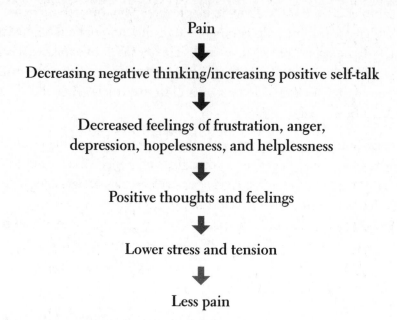

Pain

⬇

Decreasing negative thinking/increasing positive self-talk

⬇

Decreased feelings of frustration, anger,
depression, hopelessness, and helplessness

⬇

Positive thoughts and feelings

⬇

Lower stress and tension

⬇

Less pain

From Thoughts to Actions

We all move through a process from sensing and thinking to actions, and this process usually occurs at time-warp speed. Generally speaking it does not feel like a multipart process, though it is. The process is unique for each of us and is affected by many factors, but it is possible to lay out a template or outline for healthy and balanced thinking and decision making. A simplified way to represent this process is captured in the following graphic, courtesy of Johanna Franklin and Rob Hunter:

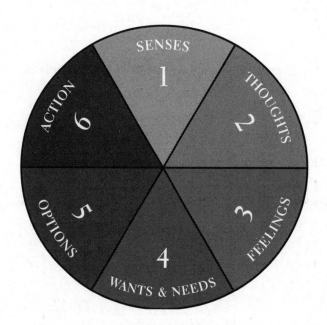

STEP ONE

Sensory perceptions: We perceive events and integrate multiple sensory inputs.

STEP TWO

Thoughts: The integrated sensory experience becomes thought—our brain generates thoughts related to what we sense, and we attach beliefs to the thoughts as to what they mean.

STEP THREE

Feelings: We feel emotions that flow from our thoughts and the beliefs we attach to them.

STEP FOUR

Wants and needs: We determine, based on our feelings, what it is we want and need relative to our specific thought(s). Step four is essentially a business plan in which we figure out what it is we need to happen.

STEP FIVE

Identify and consider options: We examine the options or choices that are open to us to get step four accomplished and select the best one with which to meet the identified needs.

STEP SIX

Take action: We implement the option/solution we determine to be the best fit for us.

When our thinking is healthy and balanced, we are progressing through these six steps on a fairly continuous basis, though most of us are not consciously aware that we're engaged in this process.

It is common for twists and inaccuracies in thinking to contribute to the train of thought becoming derailed and out of balance. When you are affected by chronic pain and/or addiction, the above process usually only includes steps one (sensing), two (thinking, typically in strictly automatic, unconscious form), and six (action). Steps three (feeling), four (considering wants and needs), and five (identifying options) are often either short-circuited or completely absent.

People with chronic pain or addiction have a tendency to avoid spending time on step three because their feeling state is so often uncomfortable. Skipping or mislabeling the feelings step makes it difficult to establish what it is we're really trying to get done (step four), and if we can't accurately identify our wants and needs, our ability to generate options that meet those needs effectively is seriously impaired. Omitting or short cutting any steps in this sequence can easily lead to imbalances in how we think.

One method we have had success with in the past is to have people visualize the brain as a muscle which has partially atrophied. That is, the "two-three-four-five" muscle group needs to be consciously taken to the mental gym and exercised. Simply getting in the habit of reminding yourself to slow your thinking down a little and make sure that you have properly identified your thoughts and feelings before deciding what needs to be achieved is a helpful skill to practice for anyone recovering from pain and/or addiction.

{ *exercise* 10.6 }

Six-Step Thought-to-Action Process _____

Take this opportunity to put this six-step process into practice. Imagine that an event or situation is being affected by your pain, and you are tempted to take medication. Apply the six steps. Focus especially on any step you might be tempted to skip. First, briefly describe the event or situation.

_____

_____

_____

_____

STEP ONE
Describe your sensory perceptions of the event.

_____

_____

_____

_____

STEP TWO
Describe the thoughts that come up for you related to this event.

_____

_____

_____

_____

STEP THREE
Describe your feelings that flow from your thoughts and beliefs related to this event.

_____

_____

_____

_____

STEP FOUR
Identify your wants and needs related to this event.

_____

_____

_____

_____

STEP FIVE
Identify the options that are available to meet your wants and needs related to this event.

_____

_____

_____

_____

Select the best option available to meet your identified needs.

_____

STEP SIX
Describe the action you will take to implement the option/solution you selected.

_____

_____

_____

_____

Dealing with Cravings

Once the drugs are stopped, you will eventually feel a lot better and may have the unrealistic expectation that you will not want to use or even think about drugs anymore. Because using drugs to relieve pain had become such a common practice, it is always possible that even as you feel better, you will think about and even crave drugs. Wanting the drug when it's absent is called craving. This does not have to be the compulsive style of "I gotta get high" that some addicts feel, but could be more like "I'm hurting and I need something to take the pain away even though it won't be good for me in the long run." This makes sense, because the pills *did relieve your pain!* So, thinking about drugs when you are in pain is not something you should feel bad or ashamed about.

If you're at this point in the book, chances are opioids didn't work for you overall. Possibly you became addicted, or the medications stopped taking the pain away but you took them anyway, or the medications caused intractable side effects, or your function decreased while you were on the medications. But if you took an opioid, it did work *in some way* to help you feel better, if only for a short while.

Now, in recovery, the negatives far outweigh the positives of using drugs, and you are committed to abstinence from opioids. That doesn't mean that you won't crave them from time to time when you are hurting physically and/or emotionally. Craving is a normal part of the process of drug dependence and recovery. Wanting relief from pain makes sense, but pain recovery consists of dealing with the pain differently. It requires your attitude to change about this short-term measure that is ineffective in the long run, so you act in a positive way and don't take the drug. Maintaining balance in pain recovery means doing your best to not use opioid pain medications, hopefully ever again.

Relapse prevention requires knowing that you are having a craving. You need to be aware of the craving so that you can take appropriate action and *not* take the drug. You must know that you are thinking about using a drug—you must bring the unconscious thought into your consciousness. After you do that, it is imperative to discuss the cravings with someone you trust who is knowledgeable. This person could be a sponsor in a twelve-step fellowship or a peer in a pain-recovery support group. It could be a health professional, counselor, or family member who understands pain recovery. Other things you can do to relieve craving include:

- Going to a meeting.

- Talking about how you were feeling before the craving occurred.

- Going for a walk or other gentle exercise (whatever will keep you busy without making your pain worse).

- Doing something kind to be helpful to someone else.

- Reading or watching a movie (preferably with someone else).

- Writing a list of the things in your life you are grateful for.

- Exploring, with a trusted person, any precipitating event, feeling, or need that might be related to that particular craving.

Cravings _____

{ *exercise* 10.7 }

Describe an episode of craving.

_____
_____
_____
_____

What actions did you take that helped diminish the craving?

_____
_____
_____
_____

What did you do that made it worse?

_____
_____
_____
_____

Write some actions you can take when you are hurting to ensure that opioids are not an option.

_____
_____
_____
_____

What If I Develop Acute Pain?

If you have a history of addiction and develop acute pain, for example, from surgery or a broken bone, then you may need to take opioids for a limited period of time. If this is the case and you can't do without them, take the smallest dose possible for as short a period of time as possible. Have someone hold and dispense the medication for you and stop as soon as you can.

Sometime in the future you may find that you have to weigh the option of taking opioid pain medications for a medical condition or procedure. First ask yourself, "Do I really need them?" Get counsel from a doctor, sponsor, and others whom you trust. Rather than deciding to take medications impulsively, slow the process down, bounce it around, write about it, pray about it in a way that makes sense to you, and explore your thoughts, emotions, body, and spirit about it.

{ *exercise* 10.8 }

Considering Medication for Acute Pain _____

Let's say the answer is that you do need to take the medication. What are the circumstances?

Surgery. If so, describe:

_____

_____

_____

_____

Injury or worsening condition. If so, describe:

_____

_____

_____

_____

Cancer or other life-threatening illness or condition. If so, describe:

_____

_____

_____

_____

Other. If so, describe:

_____

_____

_____

_____

Now think about what will be different from in the past when you used the drug. Write about your thoughts, and use the examples if applicable.

I will only use drugs for a limited period (e.g., post-op).

_____

_____

_____

_____

I'm dying and need pain relief and don't care about dependence or addiction.

_____

_____

_____

_____

I can't stand it and need relief.

_____

_____

_____

_____

Other.

_____

_____

_____

_____

If opioids reenter your central nervous system, you are in a dangerous place. We suggest you ask yourself:

What shape is your recovery in?

Physical: _____

Mental: _____

Emotional: _____

Spiritual: _____

What can you do to improve your balance and to shore yourself up against a possible relapse in the face of needing to take opioids?

_____

_____

_____

_____

_____

_____

_____

Get Into the Solution

Pain recovery is solution-based. It applies the principles of the Twelve Steps in the context of chronic pain. One of the goals of pain recovery is to help you to stop feeling like a victim of your pain. Living in pain recovery requires acceptance, hope, a positive attitude, and action. Once you can accept that you are powerless over your chronic pain, you can begin the recovery process.

Just by reading up to this point, you have taken a huge step toward pain recovery. Now it gets more difficult because the process requires you to do things that you may not want to do. However, those are often the things that are best for us—for example, going to a meeting when you don't feel like it or when your head tells you, "Not tonight, my back is hurting and I just want to lie around." Getting into the solution is learning to develop a relationship with a power greater than yourself, and being open-minded enough to consider this concept; after all, medication has been your higher power for long enough. It's trusting the process of finding a sponsor who will help you walk through the initial fear that most people experience when the anesthetic is gone. It's opening up to a counselor or therapist when you don't feel like talking. It's receiving the life-changing gifts of recovery and then giving back what was so freely given to you.

The path of healing is narrow, since changing your life takes effort and willingness, but immensely rewarding. In order to experience growth that produces change, you *must* look at yourself honestly and learn how to use the tools that will allow you to heal.

This chapter has defined the last piece of the puzzle of your pain recovery. You have seen examples of imbalance and identified actions to correct the imbalances in each of the four points. We looked, in depth, at the crucial interaction between thoughts and emotions and described how short-circuiting the process has led to imbalanced actions and behaviors. We spent some time looking at craving, and finally, at what might happen if you have acute pain that may require you to take dangerous substances.

Now it's time to sum up, consolidate your learning, and create a pain-recovery plan you will be able to follow for the rest of your life.

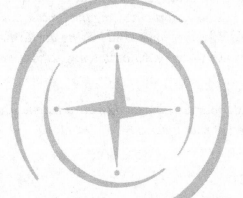

Continuing the Journey
A Long-Term Pain-Recovery Plan

Having a plan of continuing action after completing this book is essential to ensuring an ongoing healthy lifestyle in pain recovery. These next steps that you take will set the tone for your continued recovery, as well as solidify everything you have learned in the previous chapters. Please complete the following recovery plan to the best of your ability. Do not hesitate to ask others in recovery or those who are supportive of your efforts to assist in completing this plan.

Go back in this book and review the exercises you have completed. In each chapter, highlight in yellow the key things you have learned from each chapter. List these items; try to consolidate them into one phrase each.

Chapter One: **Chronic Pain**

1.

2.

3.

4.

5.

Chapter Two: Chronic Pain and Addiction

1.

2.

3.

4.

5.

Chapter Three: Am I an Addict?

1.

2.

3.

4.

5.

Chapter Four: What Is Pain Recovery?

1.

2.

3.

4.

5.

Chapter Five: Physical Balance

1.

2.

3.

4.

5.

Chapter Six: Mental Balance

1.

2.

3.

4.

5.

Chapter Seven: Emotional Balance

1.

2.

3.

4.

5.

Chapter Eight: Spiritual Balance

1.

2.

3.

4

5.

Chapter Nine: Relationships

1.

2.

3.

4.

5.

Chapter Ten: Positive Action

1.

2.

3.

4.

5.

Now prioritize these as accurately as you can—in other words, rank them from one to five in order of importance, with one being the highest importance.

List the top item from each chapter and rank those ten items in order of importance from one to ten.

1.

2.

3.

4.

5.

6.

7.

8

9.

10.

As you can see, you have a good idea of the important things you have learned from this book.

Now list concerns—these are issues that might be called "relapse triggers." Include issues that come to mind as potential trouble areas that might result in wanting to return to dysfunctional behavior patterns, including resuming drug use. Return to the previous chapters and circle problem areas in green. List at least ten here.

1.

2.

3.

4.

5.

6.

7.

8.

9.

10.

One more time, return to the text and extract or think of possible solutions for each of the potential relapse triggers. For example, when I feel afraid I will pray, call my sponsor or someone reliable, read certain pages, and write about them.

1.

2.

3.

4.

5.

6.

7.

8.

9.

10.

List specific steps that you will take to avoid relapsing when dealing with cravings, unhealthy thoughts, negative feelings, physical problems, and spiritual disconnection.

1.

2.

3.

5.

6.

7.

8.

9.

10.

BALANCE INVENTORY WORKSHEET

1. Stop and take a deep, slow breath.

2. Notice your state of each point of balance. What's going on in your body, mind, emotions, and spirit? Write your observations in the table below.

Physical	Mental	Emotional	Spiritual

3. Are these observations familiar or new? What can you compare them to?

_____

_____

_____

_____

_____

_____

_____

4. Picture your life with balance in all four points. What does it look like? What feelings does it bring up? In the table below, write about the mental picture you created of your life in balance and the feelings you have about it.

Physical	Mental	Emotional	Spiritual

5. What do you need to do in order to have the life you pictured? Set goals and create an action plan to make adjustments and changes in any areas that are imbalanced.

GOALS

1. _____

   _____

2. _____

   _____

3. _____
   _____

4. _____
   _____

5. _____
   _____

ACTION PLAN

_____
_____
_____
_____
_____

6. Contact someone from your support system and discuss what you've written.

In the event you use drugs again, what specific steps will you take to get back into the recovery process? For example, you will call a sponsor or support person and get honest, go to ninety meetings in ninety days, or seek long-term treatment if use is prolonged.

_____
_____
_____
_____
_____

Recovery Support

List the twelve-step meetings or other support groups that you are going to attend on a weekly basis (ninety meetings in ninety days is recommended for twelve-step groups).

Day	Time	Location

Appointments and Sessions

Make a list of your appointments and sessions with, for example, a counselor, psychologist, physician, or any other provider who can assist in your recovery plan.

Name	Date and Time	Type of Service

Recovery Reading and Writing Materials

List books, articles, or other materials that you will use to assist in your ongoing recovery.

_____

_____

_____

_____

_____

_____

The success of your pain recovery truly depends on how well you choose to follow this recovery plan and your willingness to do so. Recovery is a lifelong process that does not stop after completing this book; in fact, this is just beginning.

Remember that balance is a fluid, ever-changing process, so be good to yourself and make gentle, incremental changes when needed. Take this plan and post it someplace where you can look at it each and every day to remind you of the positive things that you need to do on a regular basis to stay balanced and in pain recovery.

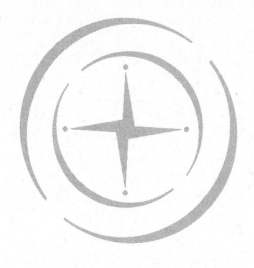

COMPANION BOOKS TO *PAIN RECOVERY*

NOW AVAILABLE

A Day without Pain

Mel Pohl, MD, FASAM with Mike Donahue

In a concise, easy-to-read format, *A Day without Pain* offers a thorough explanation for the mechanisms of pain, opioid use, and addiction, and reviews opioid-free solutions that bring relief from chronic pain.

My Pain Recovery Journal

A specialized journal designed to be compatible with *Pain Recovery* that gives those dealing with chronic pain a separate space for recording thoughts, expressing feelings, and monitoring progress. Also contains writing prompts to promote journaling that enhances the pain-recovery process.

COMING IN 2010

Pain Recovery for the Family: How to Find Balance When Someone You Love Has Chronic Pain

Chronic pain not only causes suffering and distress to those who are afflicted, it profoundly impacts the entire family. Written for family members affected by a loved one's chronic pain and substance use, this book uses an approach to healing the family that parallels the pain-recovery process for the person with chronic pain.

Facilitator's Guide for Pain Recovery

A resource for treatment professionals filled with useful tips and helpful suggestions on how to use *Pain Recovery* with chronic pain clients in a treatment setting.

Daily Meditations for Pain Recovery

Positive and inspiring messages for each day of the year help provide motivation for those trying to find balance and live in recovery from chronic pain.

To order or find more information on these and other Central Recovery Press titles, visit CentralRecoveryPress.com

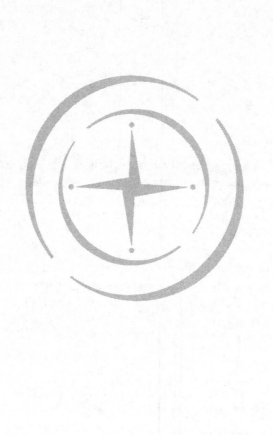

REFERENCES

Chapter One
Chronic Pain: An Overview

Farber, PL, J Blustein, E Gordon, and N Neveloff. "Pain: Ethics, Culture, and Informed Consent to Relief." *Journal of Law, Medicine & Ethics* 24, no. 4 (1996): 348–59.

National Center for Health Statistics. "Chart Book on Trends in the Health of Americans with Special Feature on Pain." In *Health, United States, 2006.* Hyattsville: CDC National Center for Health Statistics Press, 2006.

Pohl, M. *A Day without Pain.* Las Vegas: Central Recovery Press, 2008.

Society for Neuroscience. "Brain Briefings: Gender and Pain." May 2007. http://web.sfn.org/index.cfm?pagename=brainbriefings_gender_and_pain.

Chapter Two
Chronic Pain and Addiction: Double Trouble

Manchikanti, L, K Cash, K Damron, R Manchukonda, V Pampati, and C McManus. "Controlled Substance Abuse and Illicit Drug Use in Chronic Pain Patients: An Evaluation of Multiple Variables." *Pain Physician* 9 (2006):215–26.

National Institute on Drug Abuse. "Addiction is a Chronic Disease." National Institute of Health. http://www.drugabuse.gov/about/welcome/aboutdrugabuse/chronicdisease/.

National Institute on Drug Abuse. "Drugs, Brains, and Behavior - The Science of Addiction." National Institute of Health. http://www.nida.nih.gov/scienceofaddiction/index.html.

Chapter Five
Physical Balance

Barnard, N. *Foods That Fight Pain.* New York: Three Rivers Press, 1999.

Bronfort, G, M Haas, RL Evans, and LM Bouter. "Efficacy of Spinal Manipulation and Mobilization for Low Back Pain and Neck Pain: A Systematic Review and Best Evidence Synthesis." *Spine* 4, no. 3 (2004): 335–56.

Eisenberg, D, R Davis, S Ettner, S Appel, S Wilkey, M Van Rampey, and R Kessler. "Trends in Alternative Medicine Use in the United States, 1990-1997: Results of a Follow-up National Survey." *Journal of the American Medical Association* 280 (1998):1569–75.

Gagnier, JJ, MW van Tulder, BM Bermann, and C Bombardier. "Herbal Medicine for Low

Back Pain." *Cochrane Reviews* 2 (2006). http://www.cochrane.org/reviews/en/ab004504.html.

Kabat-Zinn, J. *Full Catastrophe Living.* New York: Bantam Doubleday Dell Publishing Group, Inc., 1990.

National Center for Complimentary and Alternative Medicine. "Health Topics A–Z." http://nccam.nih.gov/health/atoz.htm.

Tindle, H, R Davis, R Phillips, and D Eisenberg. "Trends in Use of Complementary and Alternative Medicine by US Adults: 1997-2002." *Alternative Therapies in Health and Medicine* 11 (2005): 42–49.

Wolsko, P, D Eisenberg, R Davis, R Kessler, and R Phillips. "Patterns and Perceptions of Care for Treatment of Back and Neck Pain: Results of a National Survey." *Spine* 28 (2003): 292–98.

Chapter Nine
Relationships

Bufalari, L, T Aprile, A Avenanti, F Di Russo, and SM Aglioti. "Empathy for Pain and Touch in the Human Somatosensory Cortex." *Cerebral Cortex* 17, no. 11 (2007): 2553–61.

Jackson, PL, A Meltzoff, and J Decety. "How Do We Perceive the Pain of Others? A Window Into the Neural Processes Involved in Empathy." *Neuroimage* 24, no. 3 (2005): 771–79.

Saarela, MV, Y Hlushchuck, AC de C Williams, M Schurmann, E Kalso, and R Hari. "The Compassionate Brain: Humans Detect Intensity of Pain from Another's Face." *Cerebral Cortex (Oxford)* 17, no 1 (2007): 230–37.

Society for Neuroscience. "Findings on Pain, Including How a Spouse Can Spur the Sense, Provide New Insights." 2002. http://www.sfn.org/index.cfm?pagename=news_11032002a.

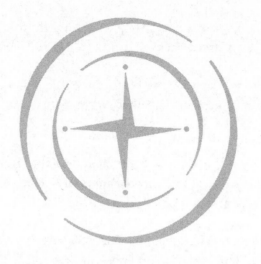

INDEX